integrated exercise

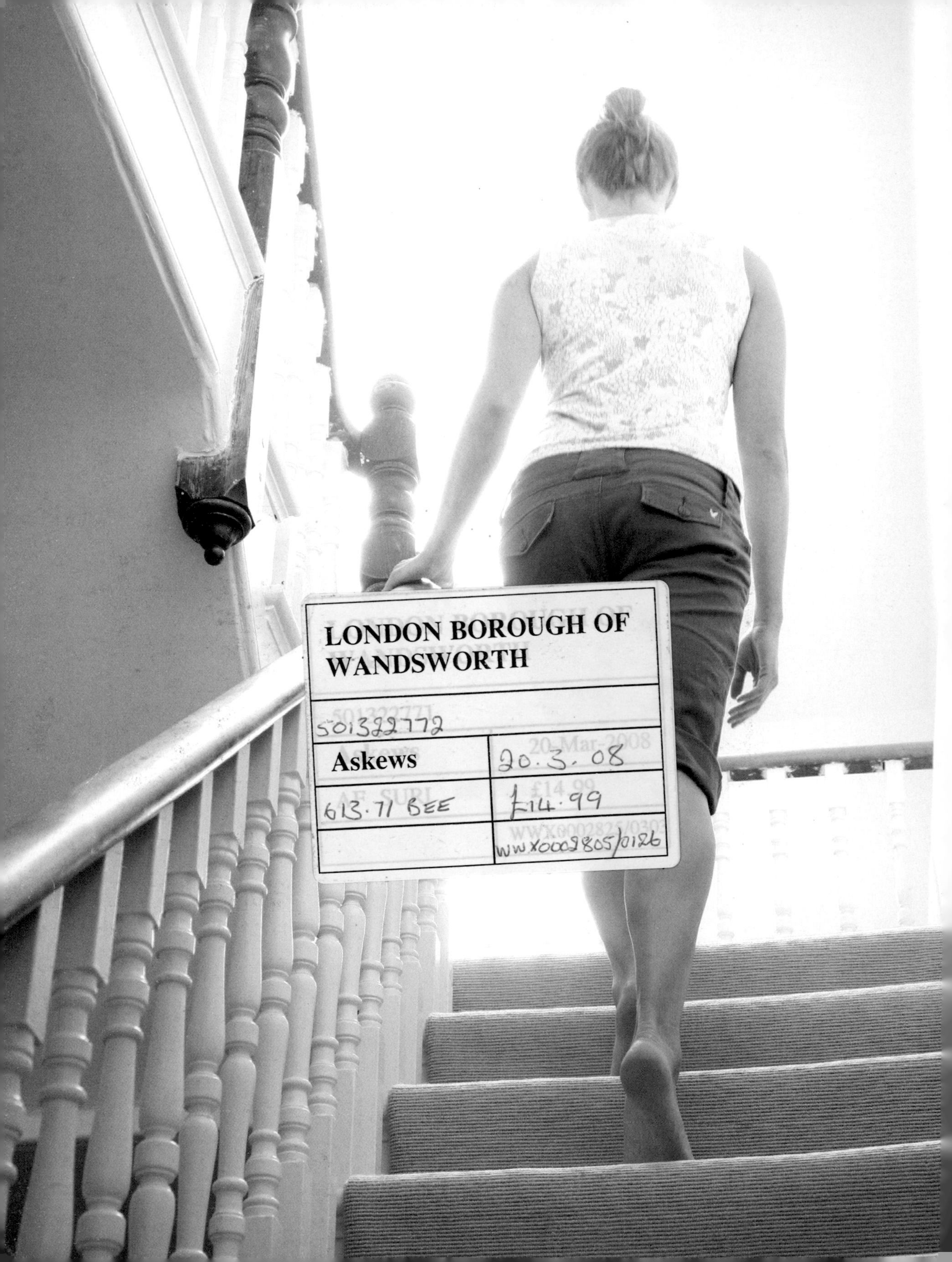

integrated exercise

How everyday activity will get you fit

Peta Bee

Kyle Cathie Limited

Frank McGrath,
may your blue eyes always sparkle.

First published in Great Britain in 2008 by
Kyle Cathie Limited
www.kylecathie.com

10 9 8 7 6 5 4 3 2 1

ISBN 978-1-85626-759-5

Text © 2008 Peta Bee
Photography © 2008 Charlie Richards
Book design © 2008 Kyle Cathie Limited

Project editor: Jennifer Wheatley
Designer: Abby Franklin
Photographer: Charlie Richards (see also below)
Copy editor: Anne Newman
Editorial assistant: Vicki Murrell
Production Director: Sha Huxtable

A Cataloguing In Publication record for this title is available from the British Library.

Printed in Singapore

acknowledgements

There are so many people who helped in the writing of this book that it is impossible to mention everyone, but my particular thanks go to:

Justine Hancock for first commissioning me to write a feature on integrated exercise in *The Times*. It set the cogs in motion for this book.

Louise Sutton of the Carnegie Faculty of Sport and Education at Leeds Metropolitan University for her support and contributions, particularly to the Integrated Eating chapter.

The many 'movers and shakers' in the fitness industry and field of sports science who have given their invaluable expertise and opinion on the text.

My super-glamorous supermodels: Simon Hammonds, Frank McGrath, Rachael Mossom, Celine and Enya Payne, Tom Richards, Grace, Michael and Eve Snelham and Laura Wheatley.

Ben, Euan, Callum and Fraser Gray for testing out many of the exercises (often inadvertently) and for being such excellent human guinea pigs.

Charlie Richards for taking such fab photographs.

Kyle Cathie, Abby Franklin, Anne Newman and Jenny Wheatley for pulling everything together so brilliantly.

Special thanks to Mum and Dad, Luci Bee, Paddy McGrath, Dearbhla McCullough and Eva Gizowska for their unconditional and unending support.

photographic acknowledgements

All photography by Charlie Richards except for the following: page 13 Laura Wheatley; 15 H. Armstrong Roberts / Corbis; 17 Ty Allison / Getty; 23 Uppercut Images / Alamy; 33–35 Olivier Blondeau / iStockphoto; 33–35 (background) iStockphoto; 42 Francesca Yorke; 43 iStockphoto; 45 Brian Carpenter / iStockphoto; 47 Stephan Kohler / iStockphoto; 57 JupiterImages / Brand X / Alamy; 79 Murat Şen / iStockphoto; 85 Randy Faris / Corbis; 86 PhotoAlto / Alamy; 87 Sean Locke / iStockphoto; 89 Chen Chun Wu / iStockphoto; 101 Francesca Yorke; 105 Greg Gerla / Alamy; 121 Florida Images / Alamy; 128 PhotoAlto / Alamy; 135 Michal Koziarski / iStockphoto; 137 image100 / Alamy; 138 PhotoAlto / Alamy; 145 Bon Appetit / Alamy; 147 Catherine dée Auvil / iStockphoto; 150 StockFood.com / Lehmann, Joerg; 156 FoodStock / Alamy; 157 (left) Shannon Long / iStockphoto (right) Peter-John Freeman / iStockphoto

contents

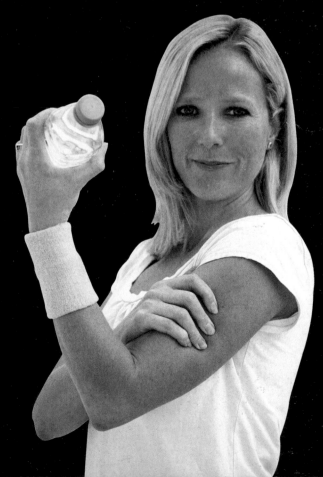

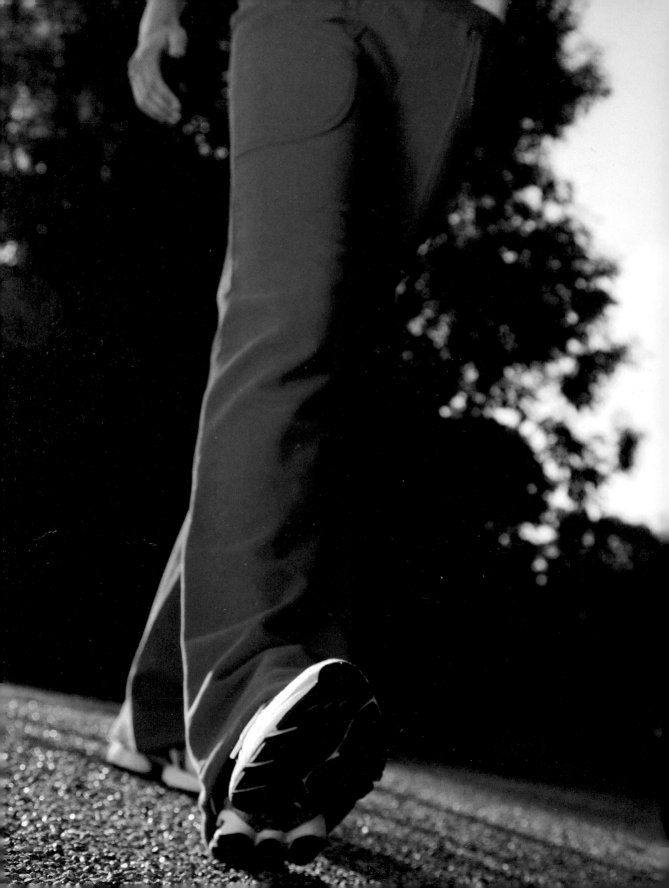

foreword

By far the most common question I am asked in a professional capacity is, 'How can I lose weight?' And the answer – which is not the one most people anticipate – is simply to get moving more often and in a greater variety of ways. Being more active should make you feel fitter, look better and provide you with more vitality and energy to go about your daily tasks. Yet the vast majority of people today lead sedentary lifestyles and their lack of physical exercise has become a serious public health concern.

Despite the very strong case presented for keeping active, many of us find it extremely difficult to incorporate physical activity or structured exercise into our daily lives, even though just thirty minutes of moderate exercise five days a week would be enough to gain health benefits. And that need not even be the kind of exercise that leaves you hot, sweaty and struggling to catch your breath. Sports physiologists have shown that moderate-intensity activity – in which your body temperature rises a little and you tax your cardio-respiratory system to the point where you are puffing but not uncontrollably – is incredibly beneficial when it comes to warding off obesity and killer illnesses such as heart disease and diabetes.

What the inactive brigade don't realise is that fitting in more exercise can be surprisingly easy. Which is where *Integrated Exercise* comes in. Written by a leading expert in the field of fitness and backed by heaps of scientific evidence, this is the definitive guide to adopting activity for life. It tackles the problems of couch- and desk-potato lifestyles and does so in a realistic way, by recognising the pressures of modern-day life in which not everybody has the time or inclination to don a leotard and do the grapevine step in aerobics.

In short, Peta Bee's plan serves to illustrate how you don't need technical equipment, a gym environment, unlimited surplus cash or extra hours in your day – all you need is some guidance, along with a dose of enthusiasm and determination.

There are infinite ways to become more active, many of which are outlined in this book; but even if you don't find the precise form of exercise to suit you in these pages, I suspect you will find the inspiration to try out something that will give you pleasure while getting you fit. Good luck in your quest to becoming a fitter, healthier and happier person. And, above all, have fun on your journey getting there.

Louise Sutton, Principal Lecturer in Health, Exercise and Nutrition at the Carnegie Faculty of Sport and Education, Leeds Metropolitan University

introduction

I am sitting in front of my keyboard, typing furiously, when the phone rings. I answer it and, as I speak, I stand up and begin pacing around the room with a sense of purpose. When the call is over, I stretch and twist my back and waist to flush out the tension created from being desk bound. Then I sit down again and begin to tap my feet on the floor and perform midriff toning exercises as I type. While working, I am also working out. That, in essence, is the underlying principle of *Integrated Exercise*.

There are a few myths about exercise that I feel should be dispelled from the outset. You don't need to be young, slim or athletic to be physically active – you just need to be motivated. And fitness should never be measured simply in terms of the calories burned, the inches whittled away or the pounds shed because its benefits are far more wide-reaching and rewarding. Physical activity need not entail expensive Lycra outfits, a personal trainer, sports drinks, muscle rubs or heart-rate monitors – it merely involves movement, preferably with gusto, but movement of any kind. Your forms of exercise can be as challenging as you want to make them – whether your aim is to walk a mile having never even walked for a bus, or to play with the children without getting breathless; the significant thing is achieving something that really matters to you.

Get real

One thing this book does not promise is to leave you with rippling muscle tone and the fitness levels of an Olympic athlete. So if you are looking for a guide to super-fitness that will see you on your way to running a marathon, completing an Iron-man triathlon or tackling the world's highest peaks then you are reading the wrong book. What you will find here, however, is sound advice, gleaned from medical, nutrition, sports science and fitness experts all over the world, that will give you the knowledge, understanding and, most importantly, the inspiration needed to become more active and therefore more healthy.

There are no rules to integrated exercise because, ultimately, only you can set them to suit your own lifestyle. Partly, it will be a journey of self-discovery, and you won't have to make any sort of huge commitment in terms of time, money or gut-busting effort along the way. Hopefully you will simply find a tip or suggestion that provides the impulse to begin moving more often and in a way that you really enjoy and that will get you started.

No need for the gym

For too many people, fitness has become synonymous with signing up to expensive gyms and fashionable fitness classes, from yogalates to punk rock aerobics. There is nothing wrong with these – or, indeed, any – approaches to becoming more active. If, in your quest to become fitter, you find that the timetable at your health club inspires you to try

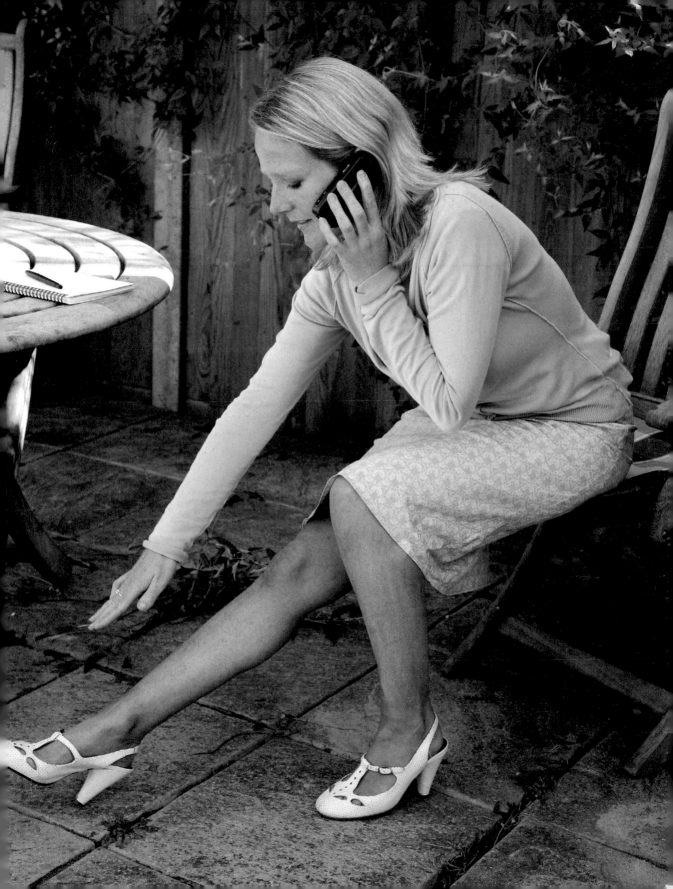

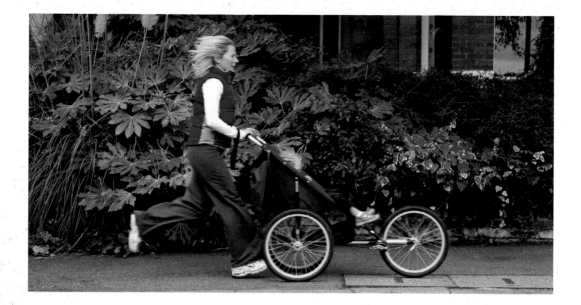

a form of exercise that makes a difference to the way you feel about yourself, then I would wholeheartedly encourage you to join up.

But gyms are not for everyone. They are certainly not for me; I have lost count of the number of times I have taken out gym memberships over the years only to lose interest after a few visits. To me, the gym environment is sterile and far from motivational. I feel self-conscious surrounded by mirrors, eagle-eyed instructors and super-skinny members of the fitterati brigade; I get exasperated by the repetition in gym classes and I can't run for more than five minutes on a treadmill without getting bored.

My most enjoyable route to fitness is to head outdoors for a long run. However, as my life has become more time crunched with children and a career eating into my day, my once- or even twice-daily run, which was usually performed in solitude along the river close to my home, is now a weekly event, if that. So with less and less time to devote solely to exercise I have had to be creative in finding ways to squeeze activity into each day.

Consequently, I arrive hot and sweaty at my son's nursery after running him there in his buggy instead of taking the car; I park at the opposite end of the high street to the local supermarket which means walking with weighted arms each time I go shopping; I run (rather than plod) up and down stairs several times a day; and I power-walk my dog at a much faster pace than I ever did before.

With *Integrated Exercise,* you will learn through trial and error what works for you. I have developed my own recipe for success, based on the top ten principles opposite. You may find these points helpful or you may discover entirely different affirmations of your own. What matters is that they are convenient, practical and manageable for the way you live your life.

Finally, let me leave you with a thought. In the few minutes it took you to read these pages, you will have expended about 5 calories if sitting, fewer if you were lying down. Had you been walking, you could multiply that figure by at least two. Now, don't you wish you'd read them while marching on the spot?

my top ten ways to successfully integrate exercise

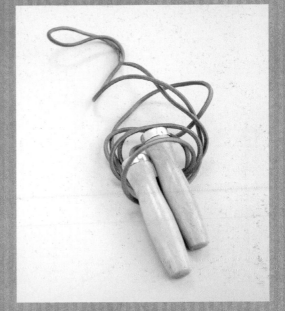

1 Never take the car when you could walk or run the journey in question.

2 When walking, do so at a pace where you feel you might break into a run if you were to go any faster.

3 Never use a lift unless there is no alternative.

4 Take the stairs rather than an escalator whenever possible; if an escalator is the only option, power-walk up the moving steps.

5 Never use the moving walkways – set yourself a challenge to reach the furthest end before those who take the lazy route.

6 Stand up on short train and bus journeys and on longer ones make sure you stand up or walk about at least every fifteen minutes.

7 Do something active every time you get up to make a coffee (which, in my case, is often) – you could run up the stairs, put the washing out, unload the dishwasher or clean a window, for example.

8 If you have children, encourage them to integrate exercise too. Don't buy them games involving nothing but twiddling knobs on a console. Engage them in your active lifestyle. Go for walks, buy them footballs, basketball nets and skipping ropes – anything that will help them to appreciate that sport and activity are enjoyable. Play with them whenever you can; the more active you are, the more they will be too (and vice versa).

9 Set yourself mini fitness challenges. If you are walking to the shops try alternating fast and slow walking or weaving between lamp posts.

10 Put extra effort into every household chore. The end result – a stronger, fitter you – will make it well worth the extra elbow grease.

chapter one

integrated exercise for life

Being fat and unfit were not always issues for mankind; it's not that long ago that weight problems were an affliction of the minority. Integrating exercise into their daily lives was something our older relatives and our ancestors took for granted. And in the very distant past, there was little time for sloth: survival depended on hunting and gathering for food and all the running around that entailed meant that cavemen simply didn't get fat.

Changes to this frenetic means of survival came gradually. Eventually our ancestors discovered how to breed animals and cultivate crops without having to roam miles for food, but their daily lives were still a strenuous grind. Then, in the 1800s, the Industrial Revolution brought the technological advances that would alter employment and lifestyle patterns beyond recognition. But it was not until fifty years ago that we really began our descent towards indolence. In the 1950s, daily levels of physical activity were equivalent to walking three to five miles; today the average person fails to cover that distance in a week.

In Europe, the incidence of obesity has almost trebled since the 1980s with half of the adult population and more than 21 million children now classified as overweight or obese; in America, 64.5 per cent of adults are overweight or obese, a figure that is set to rise to 73 per cent by 2010.

The repercussions of this epidemic are alarming. As we wobble our way through life, our chances of suffering an illness for which fatness is a major risk factor – diabetes, heart disease, stroke and cancer – are higher than ever. And the main reason why waistlines are expanding so rapidly? Inertia.

The cost of convenience

What we have gained in convenience from labour-saving devices over the last half century, we have paid for in terms of a sharp decline in physical activity. We use cars, buses or trains to get to work; our children are driven to school; escalators and lifts have replaced conventional stairs in shopping centres and office blocks and flats. Washing machines, vacuum cleaners, dishwashers and electric lawnmowers all minimise the effort required to maintain a clean and tidy home. And the upshot is that almost one third of adults spend over ten hours sitting down every day, adding up to a staggering average of thirty-two years and four months of their expected life span.

The TV trap

Television has us tethered to the sofa, cars have replaced walking or cycling and more and more time is being spent slumped over computers than doing household chores. Researchers have linked these twenty-first-century habits directly with obesity and its related health problems. It has been proven time and again, for instance, that the more television someone watches, the fatter they get and that those people who watched a lot of television as children are more likely to be overweight as adults.

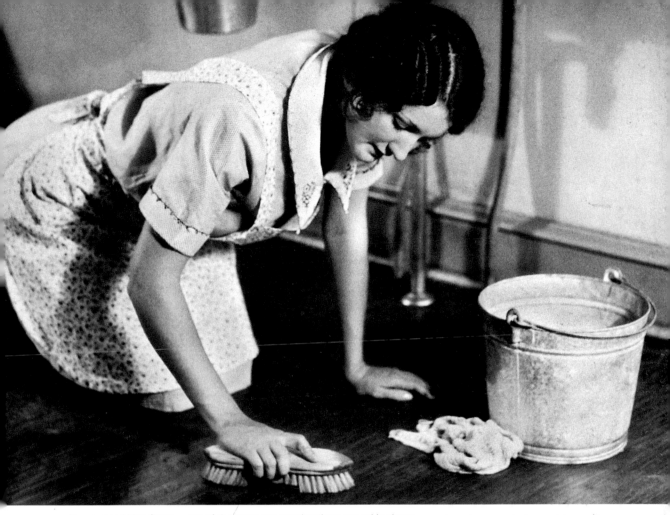

Above: scrubbing floors – one of the ways our grandmothers stayed in shape.

Reports on both sides of the Atlantic confirm that the majority of people are now not active enough to benefit their health. A government survey in the UK suggests that as many as three in four women and three in five men lead such sedentary lives that they are putting their health at risk. Even people who report they work out often don't do as much physical activity as they claim. Scientists found that while 47 per cent of people who were asked to record their exercise patterns over seven days suggested they had exercised moderately during that period, only 15 per cent had pushed themselves to a level that met researchers' definition of moderate activity.

Of course, our diets have changed, too. Consumption of fruit and vegetables falls well below the 'five a day' recommended by nutritionists and instead we gobble too many fat- and calorie-laden sugary snacks. But while it is easy to blame weight gain in the West on an increasing intake of fast food and fatty snacks – and, admittedly, it hasn't helped matters – people today actually consume fewer calories, not more when compared with what was eaten in the 1960s. The main reason for our fatness is high levels of inactivity.

the gym conundrum

One of the apparent paradoxes of the weight gain epidemic is that it is happening at a time when so many people are joining gyms and health clubs. Around one in eight people is now a member of a private gym or health club and memberships have increased every year since the initial boom of the early 1980s when Jane Fonda was urging us all to pull on the leggings and go for the burn. So if more of us are paying up to plod on a treadmill or take part in an aerobics class, why are obesity statistics still rising?

There is no straightforward answer, although my personal hunch (and that of some researchers) is that while gyms do have their place in society and certainly help many to reach supreme levels of fitness and improved body image, it is often the case that they can sustain people's enthusiasm and motivation for a limited period only. Some psychologists say that for many people the clinical environment and image-conscious atmosphere of the gym are enough to put many people off working out altogether. Also, many of those who fork out the money to join a gym soon find its institutionalised exercise format similar to embarking on a strict diet or detox programme: it presents a means to an end but is difficult to stick to in the long term.

One report found that a fifth of members work out in their gym once a month or even less frequently, burning what amounts to an average of around 100–200 calories a week there – less than they would use on a brisk weekly walk. In reality, only 20–25 per cent of paid-up gym members regularly attend, and those who do spend much of their time chatting to others, getting drinks or wandering between equipment. Some consumer surveys put the gym dropout rate at more than 80 per cent within the first eight weeks of signing up.

Even among those who do work out regularly at the gym, there is evidence that it might not be the most beneficial approach. Three-quarters of gym members schedule their visits to coincide with a specific television

> ### did you know?
> Celebrities are catching on to the idea that slotting more activity into their hectic schedules is as effective as taking time out to visit a gym. Victoria Beckham told GMTV how 'running after three children' is enough to keep her in super-slim shape. And, in a magazine interview, Hollywood actress Sharon Stone gave integrated exercise her seal of approval: 'I still do push-ups and sit-ups,' she said, 'but I also try to do things such as walking up the stairs, and not taking a lift. I'll also park my car farther away from a store so I have to walk a few steps more. If you keep it up over a long period, you don't have to do too much.'

programme, one survey found. Studying the habits of gym-goers, psychologists reported that many become so engrossed in watching TV that they simply go through the motions of exercise – slowly pedalling or inching along on the treadmill – and barely breaking sweat.

In a study in the Netherlands of healthy, non-obese adults, it was found that people who spend more time doing moderate, integrated-style exercise burned more calories than those who performed shorter, sharper workouts. Why? Because after a hard morning or lunchtime workout, people typically limit their physical activity for the rest of the day.

Gyms only work if you use them well and the reality is that most people don't.

workout

Breakfast cereals have a wholesome image, but be careful to check the nutritional labels, even those marketed for children. A typical sweetened rice-based cereal provides 24 per cent of the daily sugar intake recommended for five-to-ten year olds in a 30g serving (a small bowl). With 174 calories in a bowl and 40g of sugar that's hardly a healthy option and to burn it off you'd need to do one of the following:

- ice skate for 50 minutes
- do light weight training for 42 minutes
- take part in some vigorous football-supporting for 45 minutes
- star jumps for 22 minutes
- boxing for 18 minutes.

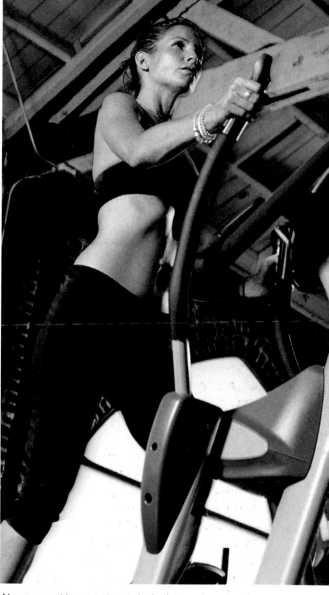

Above: repetition at gyms can be boring.

strange but true

Gym subscriptions were identified by one online bank as one of the direct-debit payments customers most frequently forget to cancel when they no longer use the facilities.

What makes integrated exercise different from other fitness programmes is that you decide which activity to do, when to do it and for how long – it can be whatever you want it to be. There is no bewildering fitness jargon to decipher, no need for personal trainers or to wear tight-fitting Lycra and no prescriptive schedules to stick to. Anything that gets your muscles working, your joints moving and your heart pumping faster can be considered integrated exercise. And, as you will discover further into this book, that can be anything from dusting to dog-walking. All that really matters is whether it works for you.

As a firm convert to this approach to activity, I could fill page after page telling you how it has helped me (and many people I know who unwittingly practise integrated exercise) to stay fit, reasonably slim and, most rewarding of all, in tip-top health most of the time. But don't just take my word for it; integrated exercise – billed to become one of the hottest fitness trends by the *New York Times* and *Los Angeles Times* – is based on scientific fact. Experts are now lining up to extol the benefits of the approach: the US Centers for Disease Control and Prevention and the American College of Sports Medicine have already produced a chart showing the calorie-burning effects of daily activities. Likewise, British, American and Australian governments all back the concept of integrating exercise into your day through gardening, carrying shopping bags or walking the dog in small, regular bursts over twenty-four hours for improved overall health.

A fitness trend we can all love

One of the reasons why integrated exercise works is because it is easy to do with some consistency. That is helpful when it comes to burning calories and getting fitter, but has wider-reaching benefits too. Sports scientists have discovered that tough sessions of aerobic exercise releases damaging free radicals in previously sedentary and unfit people, thereby damaging their health. Such exercise is the kind which involves taking the heart rate to approximately 85 per cent of its maximum for more than 10 minutes and which leaves you seriously breathless and sweaty. With integrated exercise the effort required is less extreme (you should be puffed, but not exhausted when you are doing it) and, according to this theory, the free radical damage is minimal.

Even experts who preached the benefits of gyms and aerobics during the late 1970s and 80s now acknowledge that they were wrong to tell people that prolonged, continuous exercise and 'going for the burn' were the only ways to get fit. They include Harvey Simon, an associate professor of medicine at Harvard Medical School, who now concedes that anything that gets you moving – from gardening to sex – can and will contribute to your health.

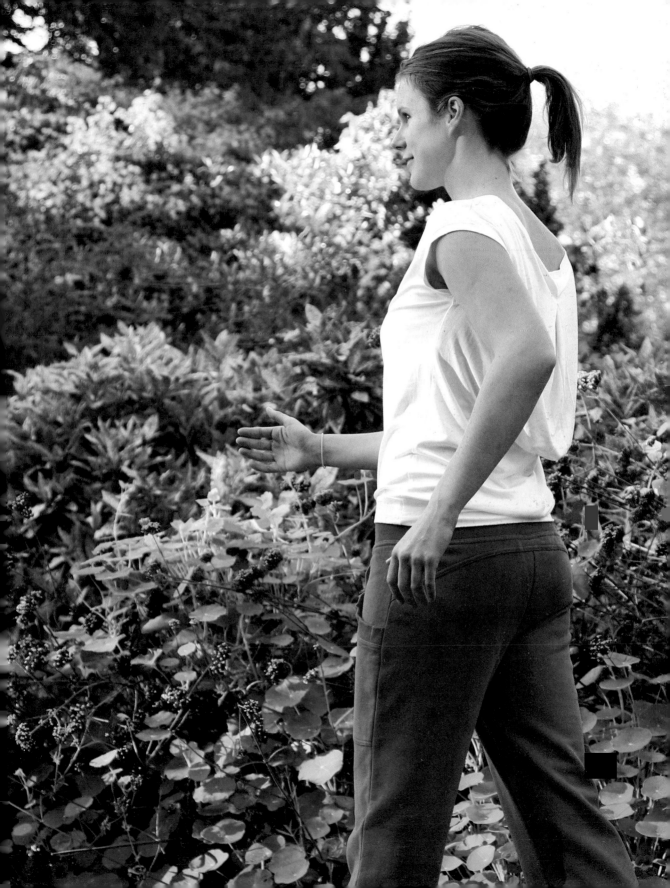

It is always far easier to think of reasons not to become more active than to bite the bullet and get moving. But the longer you procrastinate, the more of a barrier exercise becomes in your own mind. Do you think you have valid reasons not to integrate exercise into your life? Well, if any of these is one of them, think again.

'I don't have time'

The beauty of integrated exercise is that you do not need to set time aside to do it. Simply carry on with your regular daily routine, but insert slots of activity when you might previously have been inert. Walk to the shops instead of taking a car; climb the stairs instead of taking a lift; do the housework yourself instead of employing a cleaner. The important thing to remember is that every second you are active makes a difference.

'I can't afford it'

Integrating exercise costs absolutely nothing. There are no fancy equipment, no membership fees and no travel expenses. Should you wish to progress, there are things you can buy to help you (such as comfortable trainers, a good skipping rope or a pedometer) but these are not essential. Improvising with every-day household items is equally as effective.

'It's boring'

This is, perhaps, the lamest excuse of all. With this route to improved fitness, you are in charge of how much, how little and what type of exercise you do. By the time you have read this book you will be brimful of ideas for how to make your own integrated plan work for you.

'I'm too old'

Age is not an issue when it comes to integrating exercise into your life. If you have been sedentary for a prolonged period of time or if you suffer from a degenerative condition, then it is recommended you seek advice from your doctor before embarking on any form of activity. But integrating activity into your daily life has many advantages for the illnesses and complaints commonly linked to old age (see pages 22 and 23) and research confirms it's never too late to make amends. One of the integrative exercisers I admired most was my great-auntie Eve who incorporated a daily walk to and around the shops for the last few decades of her life until just a few months before she passed away, aged 101.

'I'm too overweight'

One of the truisms of exercise is that the most difficult part is hurdling the psychological barrier. For people who consider themselves overweight, this is particularly pertinent – it is all too easy to underestimate the amount of psychological gusto it takes to raise yourself from an armchair to walk up the stairs a few times or around the block when you feel too heavy. But the first step is the hardest and from that point on your attitude will change due to the fact that you have already achieved something. Bite the bullet and do something for yourself – I promise you won't regret it.

ten great reasons to integrate exercise every day

1 Raise your self-image: the most important thing to consider when you embark on your integrated exercise plan is that you are doing it for the right reasons. And, as with any fitness regimen, that means doing it for yourself and nobody else. Initially, your goals might be cosmetic – you may want to lose weight or get rid of your flabby underarms. But when you start to exercise more, the focus will shift from what your body looks like to how it can perform. You will marvel at the way your body responds and reacts to physical activity and your self-esteem and body image will soar. Studies have shown that active people do not have the same levels of body insecurity as couch potatoes. In fact, they are more self-confident, better at setting goals and meeting them and more likely to have successful careers. Let that be you.

2 Ward off arthritis: exercise has been shown to reduce the debilitating pain caused by arthritis and to delay arthritic disability. Yet studies in the UK and USA found that many people with this condition shy away from activity in the mistaken belief it will worsen their suffering. A little exercise often is what is recommended to help people with arthritis to become stronger and more mobile. That makes integrated exercise the perfect choice. Talk to your GP before embarking on any type of exercise plan, but the chances are that 'little and often' will be the way forward.

3 Strengthen your bones: the bone-thinning disease, osteoporosis, will affect one in three women and one in twelve men at some time in their lives. Known as the silent epidemic because people don't realise they have the disease until they suffer a fracture, osteoporosis is caused by the loss of bone calcium at a greater rate than it is replaced, resulting in fragile and porous bones. Activities in which the body weight is supported (such as swimming and cycling) do not have significant strengthening effects on bones, but weight-bearing exercises (in which you support your own body weight) are excellent bone builders. Walking and jogging, performing star jumps, skipping or resistance work (such as digging or carrying your shopping) are ideal. According to the National Osteoporosis Society, research shows that just fifteen skips a day can make a significant difference. Taking the stairs instead of a lift also helps. Running upstairs provides an average of twenty beneficial, high-impact jolts to the spine and hips. Do this five times a day and those hundred jolts will protect your skeleton.

4 Boost your brainpower: as we get older, blood flow to the brain slowly decreases and brain cells shrink in size. But, remarkably, exercise can help to halt this process. Gentle aerobic activity increases oxygen supply to the brain, helping it to become more alert and efficient. Regular activity was found by researchers to have a direct influence on the mental tasks controlled by the frontal and prefrontal cortex – the brain parts responsible for planning and memory among other vital functions. Elderly people who remain physically active are much less likely to develop Alzheimer's disease or other declines in mental ability. Researchers who monitored 2,288 people over the age of 65 concluded that there is a close link between mind and body in old age and that physical and mental performance go hand in hand.

5 **Relieve stress:** exercise is more than just a means of sweating away calories you have consumed. It literally gobbles up the adverse effects of pent-up tension and boosts blood levels of beta-endorphins, the naturally occurring opiates that can relieve stress and heighten our mood. Other nerve chemicals like adrenaline, serotonin and dopamine, all of which are required to produce a feeling of euphoria, are secreted in the brain during exercise. Even if all you manage to squeeze into your day is a short stroll to the shops, you can still expect immediate psychological gains. One study found a ten-minute walk left subjects feeling more relaxed and energetic.

6 **Ward off heart disease:** there is little doubt that a lack of exercise is a major factor in increasing the risk of death from heart disease. Findings from the British Heart Foundation (BHF) show that as many as two out of five deaths from heart disease in women are due to a lack of physical activity. As a consequence, the BHF does not recommend taking up squash, tennis or any other physically demanding sport, but rather to integrate activities such as walking to and from the station or shops to get in a half hour of daily activity. The foundation has launched a major campaign called '30-a-day' (see page 160) to encourage the over-fifties to integrate activity into their daily life. There are other heart benefits to being more active. Walking three times a week can slow down the progression of peripheral artery disease (PAD), a condition that involves hardening of the blood vessels in the legs and elsewhere. PAD affects around 20 per cent of the elderly population and often causes a sharp decline in movement ability. Researchers looked at the exercise habits of 417 men and women with the condition and found that those who walked three or more times a week showed a significantly smaller annual decline in the distance walked in 6 minutes.

7 **Lower the risk of cancer:** it is well documented that people who lead active lifestyles are less at risk of getting cancer, a link experts think is probably due to positive hormonal and metabolic changes that occur when a person is active. One study involving 832 women with endometrial cancer and a control population who didn't have the disease found that women who integrated exercises like household chores and walking into their lives were at a 30 per cent lower risk of getting the disease. Another study showed that the risk of death among women who had breast cancer was up to 54 per cent less in those who were active every day. Perhaps most inspiring were the results of a study of more than 200,000 women from nine European countries; it found that doing household chores regularly was far more cancer protective than occasionally playing intensely demanding sport. Housework cut breast cancer risk by 30 per cent among pre-menopausal and by 20 per cent among post-menopausal women tested.

8 **Increase your libido:** not only is sexercise a great way to integrate activity into your life (see page 118), but general exercise is among the best ways to boost your sex life. Countless studies have demonstrated the way regular activity can boost your libido. When seventy-eight healthy

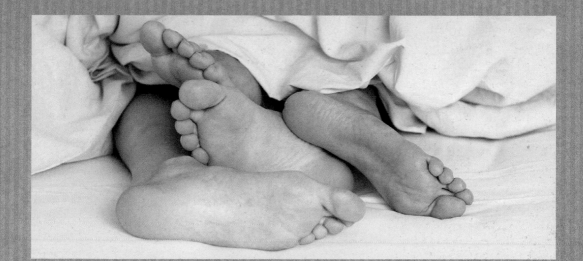

but sedentary middle-aged men were assigned a gentle activity programme, the former couch potatoes reported more reliable sexual functioning, more frequent sexual activity and orgasms and greater satisfaction during sex. Other researchers have shown how exercise can help reduce the incidence of erectile dysfunction and impotence in men. Regular activity also boosts feelings of sexual attractiveness, in turn improving sexual performance and satisfaction.

9 **Beat depression:** researchers reported that three brisk 30-minute walks each week were more effective in reducing depression than drugs from the same family as Prozac. Six months after their 156 subjects had completed the 16-week study, only 8 per cent of the exercisers saw their depression return. Other studies have shown that a short stroll or half an hour of gentle activity provided an instant lift for the moderately depressed, giving them the same sort of mental 'pick-me-up' they might normally have got from cigarettes, coffee or binge-eating. They also felt less tense, angry and tired.

10 **Change your body shape:** undoubtedly, integrating more exercise into your life will mean more calories burned and – provided you eat the same amount or less – weight loss. And, because it is so varied, it utilises many different muscles and involves the body moving in different directions across different planes – to a far greater degree than you are likely to achieve in the average gym session. Changing activities regularly also means that more of these muscles will be worked harder so that they lose the layer of fat that might initially lie over them to reveal a more toned body. Do not be mistaken – integrated exercise alone will never give you the fitness levels or chiselled physique of a top athlete. But the more active you are, the more lean tissue will replace fatty and the closer you will be to looking and feeling healthy.

the science

While blinding you with science is not what this book is about, it is important to have a little knowledge on just why integrated exercise is so helpful and, not least, the following fact:

When calories expended exceed calories consumed, you will lose weight.

A 'NEAT' reason to integrate exercise

For any exercise or diet plan to be successful in terms of weight loss and shaping up, it must have the above maxim as its underlying principle. No approach – no matter what claims it makes – will work unless it steers you towards burning more calories through physical activity than you obtain from food.

In that respect, integrated exercise is no different. But emerging research confirms that the type of exercise you can slip into your day is particularly effective in winning the battle of the bulge. In the most detailed study ever of integrated-style exercise a team of scientists at the renowned Mayo Clinic in Minnesota found that lean people perform low-grade, mundane bodily movements – such as general fidgeting, standing up then sitting down, tapping their toes or twiddling their thumbs – far more often than obese individuals. In fact, overweight people in the studies spent 2

hours longer each day sitting down, while the extra movements made by lean people were enough to burn around 350 calories a day which could add up to a weight loss of between 10 and 30 pounds a year. Experts have now coined a phrase for this incidental movement, calling it NEAT (non-exercise activity thermogenesis), and they consider it a more important factor than strenuous exercise in determining who is destined to become obese or overweight.

did you know?
Regular activity can boost the body's rate of wound-healing, a process that normally slows down with age.

Researchers gave each of twenty-eight participants a small puncture wound to the back of their upper arm. Half of the subjects had started exercising three or four times a week about a month before the study, while the rest were inactive. Results showed that the skin wounds healed, on average, ten days faster in those who were active. The results are significant because the quicker a wound heals, the less chance there is of it becoming infected.

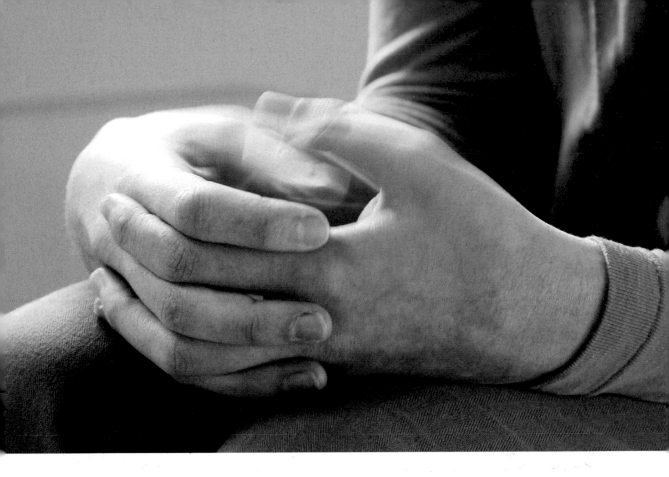

Keep fidgeting

It is now accepted that NEAT plays such a considerable role in the gobbling up of calories during daily life that the US Department of Health and Social Services is one of the organisations encouraging people to move about, fidget and become more restless more often. In one of their studies, the Mayo Clinic team followed ten men and ten women, not all of them overweight but who all considered themselves to be couch potatoes. They were asked to wear high-tech clothing for 24 hours a day over 10 days. Sensors on the garments could detect the merest twiddle of a thumb in measurements taken every half a second. The study found that leaner people spent at least 150 more minutes moving their bodies in some way.

The bad news for more sedentary individuals is that their tendency towards a couch potato existence is probably genetic. The results of the Mayo Clinic research appear to indicate that thinner people are often born with a propensity to move about more and that those prone to piling on the pounds need to make a conscious effort to be more active. Even after they have lost weight, formerly obese people are inherently inclined to sit still for longer periods than their naturally slim counterparts.

But the good news is that integrated exercise increases NEAT and overall energy expenditure whatever your genetic make-up. With a little focused effort, your energy balance can be shifted and you will watch the weight drop off.

super-fit,
not super-skinny

A mistake so often made is to assume that the primary goal of exercise should be to attain a super-skinny physique. It is far better to be a little bit rounded and a regular exerciser than to be rake-thin but unfit.

It is well documented that people who exercise consistently and often are healthier overall. Those who are slim but do not exercise are still prone to raised levels of cholesterol, insulin and C-reactive protein (a substance considered a risk factor for heart disease) – all markers for a shorter, lower quality, life.

Exercise physiologists are leading the way to a better understanding of weight and fitness. They now know that activity has a powerful effect on health, no matter how fat or thin you are. Looking at levels of C-reactive protein in a group of young men, physiologists found the lowest readings were recorded in those who exercised most often, regardless of their weight. Fit but fat diabetics have also been found to be less likely to die from their condition than their thin, unfit counterparts.

work it out

A yoghurt might seem like the low-fat dieter's dream snack, but make sure you check the label – some desserts in the chill cabinet are anything but healthy. While the label boasts 'Virtually fat free' they can be very highly sweetened – with fructose, artificial sweeteners and even crushed cake pieces. Some yoghurt-based treats contain 120 calories per individual pot and 9.6g of sugar per 100g. To burn that off you'd need to do one of the following:

- take up and re-lay carpets for 20 minutes
- scrape off wallpaper for 30 minutes
- walk while carrying books back to the library for 18 minutes
- weed the garden for 26 minutes
- groom a dog for 30 minutes.

how integrated exercise helps to regulate your appetite

Start following the integrated plan and you could find you eat less as a result. People who work out diligently at the gym, putting in considerable effort on the treadmill, stepper or exercise activity of their choice could be left sweating and panting in vain.

Studies have found that the harder the workout attempted, the more calories women (and this particular anomaly seems peculiar to females) are likely consume when it is over. In one study of thirteen fit, lean women, subjects were invited to eat as much as they wanted at a buffet lunch following a morning gym session. They also had access to an unlimited number of snacks. It was found that those who pushed themselves to the limit in high-intensity workouts, such as running at a pace too fast to hold a conversation, were so hungry when they finished that they gobbled up in excess of 90 per cent of the calories they had just burned. Most of the 878 calories the women ingested came from fat.

Conversely, those individuals who adopted a more leisurely approach in a low to moderate integrated style of exercise replaced only around one-third of the calories they had used up when their exercise session was completed.

Although there is always a slight shift in metabolism after physical activity, this does not account for the excess food eaten after a tough workout. The findings of the study suggested that, in the knowledge they had completed a virtuous workout, the women simply could not resist the temptation to eat.

A more relaxed approach to exercise results in faster weight loss in the long term.

did you know?

You can integrate exercise for the mind as well as the body. Psychiatrists have studied problem-solving games such as crosswords, Scrabble and Sudoku, and say that, if practised regularly along with physical exercise, these mind-stretchers help to keep the brain cells active and healthy. Playing such games every day can make a difference to how your brain works. In a small study, eight people were assigned to problem-solving activities while nine continued their regular routine. Brain scans showed that those following the 'brain bootcamp' regime developed significantly more efficient cell activity on the left side of the brain, in the area crucial for verbal memory and controlling everyday tasks. They also reported being less forgetful and had slightly better objective memory scores than the control group.

what is the meaning of 'fitness'?

Fitness is a word that is so often bandied around, but we rarely stop to think what it actually means. In fact, defining fitness is not easy, simply because there are many different levels of fitness and being fit means different things to different people. In a broad sense, to be fit requires the use of a range of muscles and physiological functions in a huge variety of ways. And just as there is no magic recipe to get someone fit overnight, so there is no single form of exercise that will result in total, all-round fitness.

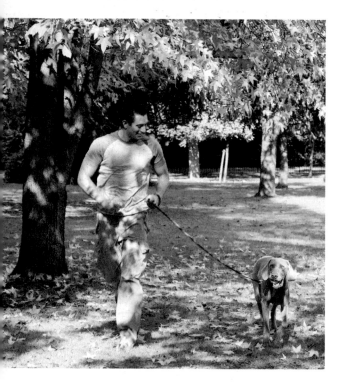

Take top sports people. All of those at the pinnacle of their game are supremely fit. Even so, their fitness is usually specific to their sport – their particular strengths from years of training are not directly transferable to another activity. Yes, they would probably be fitter than the average person in all respects, but a professional runner would not possess the kind of fitness required to compete at Wimbledon, for example, just as a top golfer would struggle to run a marathon or swim the Channel.

So, before you embark on integrated exercise, ask yourself what fitness means to you. For most people reading this book, the aim is probably to achieve a level of fitness that will put an end to being overweight, feeling tired and constantly stressed. You probably want to look better, feel better and have more energy to expend on fun, every-day activities and still have some energy left at the end of the day.

When you attain that level and can see and feel the benefits, you may want to consider more ambitious fitness goals, such as completing a fun run or triathlon or even taking up a radically different sport. I like to think of fitness as being a continuum – there are always new things to try, and new ways to challenge your body and mind. What is important, however, is that it is you and nobody else who decides when and how to push your body through barriers, whether that means progressing from a walk to a jog or from a train journey to a bike ride.

formulating an exercise plan

Whatever your aspirations, the basics of any programme should incorporate three elements: aerobic exercise, strength/resistance work and flexibility.

Aerobic exercise

This should be the mainstay of any activity plan and includes any exercise that requires the body to increase its use of oxygen. While running, swimming and cycling are among the most effective means of achieving this, aerobic activity can encompass everything from skipping to fast pram pushing or from walking up stairs to speedy inline skating.

But how does aerobic exercise benefit the body? Well, when you exercise aerobically your muscles need to use more oxygen than they would if you were standing still. The heart responds by pumping more blood which carries oxygen around the body. At first, this feels like hard work, but the more aerobic activity you do, the more efficient your body becomes at using the oxygen supplies available. In due course, the cardiovascular system also improves so that the heart can accomplish more work in the same time.

Within months of becoming more aerobically active, your resting heart rate – the average number of heartbeats a minute – will drop. This is a sign that your heart is pumping more powerfully than before and that both your heart and lungs are working more efficiently. It is also considered that, in conjunction with a healthy diet (see Chapter 9), aerobic activity is the best route to reducing body fat and boosting your metabolism – do it regularly and your body literally gobbles up calories at a faster rate.

In practical terms, increased amounts of aerobic activity mean that your life will become more pleasurable. With a strong heart and healthy lungs you will be able to run for a bus without gasping for breath, play more energetically with the grandchildren when you get older and climb up the stairs without having to sit down at the top!

Your mind will benefit too – physiologists have shown that any type of aerobic activity results in the release of feel-good hormones called endorphins that flood into your bloodstream, leaving you in a better mood. What could be better than that?

Integrated aerobic exercises include:

- Cycling (see page 97)
- Running/jogging (see page 98)
- Walking (see page 91)
- Nordic walking (see page 90)
- In-line skating (see page 102)
- Skipping (see page 130)
- Step/stair climbing (see page 38)
- Dog walking (see page 70)
- Strollercise (see page 111)
- Giving piggy backs (see page 115)
- Mallercise (see page 84)
- Sea-walking (see page 138)
- Pedalo (see page 139)
- Vigorous dancing (see page 110)

Strength/resistance exercise

Contrary to popular belief, strength exercises do not begin and end in the gym or weights room. Nor does working towards getting stronger muscles mean you end up looking like the Incredible Hulk. A completely diverse range of integrated activities will build muscle strength and improve muscle tone and can be performed anywhere – from the supermarket to the garden.

Most of the latest research shows that the quickest way to lose weight and keep it off is to incorporate aerobic exercise (see page 29) with some strength or resistance activities. Adding muscle mass through this type of exercise can help overweight people move faster so they burn more calories. Stronger muscles mean more lean muscle mass and less fatty tissue; metabolically active muscle tissue burns calories at a faster rate.

One study found that strength-based exercises just twice a week helped women ward off the tummy fat that can accumulate in middle age. And it has been shown that lifting weighty objects can boost your self-image.

Integrated resistance/strength-based exercises include:

- Gardening (see page 72)
- Shopping (see page 84)
- Supermarket workout (see page 80)
- Baby-flexing (see page 106)
- Giving piggy backs (see page 115)
- Leapfrogs (see page 127)
- Sofacise (see page 64 onwards)
- Hotel-room workout (see page 140)
- DIY (see page 77)
- Sexercise (see page 118)

Flexibility

Often referred to as stretching, it is sometimes wrongly assumed that flexibility exercises are needed only during warm-up and cool-down routines pre- and post-workout. Actually, good flexibility is required to perform a wide range of daily chores and, as such, is a vital part of all-round body health and fitness.

One thing stretching does not do is burn calories at a fast rate, but it serves important functions. Its primary role is to lengthen muscles and increase the range of movement around a joint. That, in turn, makes the body less vulnerable to injuries such as strains and muscle pulls and less likely to develop the kind of poor posture that leads to back pain.

Keeping flexible is particularly important as you get older. With age and inactivity our range of motion decreases to the extent that reaching to get something off the top shelf of a cupboard might, eventually, test this range beyond its comfort zone.

There are hundreds of ways to stretch and you may have some favourites that you wish to incorporate into your daily integrated regime. But even if all you did was to stand up at your desk and stretch your arms into the air once an hour, the benefits would be profound.

Integrated flexibility exercises include:

- Housework-out (see page 58)
- Deskercise (see page 47)
- Plane/train exercises (see page 136)
- Fidgeting (see page 25)
- Supermarket workout (see page 80)
- Sofacise (see page 63)
- Gardening workout (see page 72)

getting started: executing your plan

One of the hardest things about getting fit is simply getting started – particularly when you think that might involve devoting huge chunks of your day to exercise. Integrating exercise into your day, however, means precisely that – your workout is cleverly incorporated into your daily routine and there is no need to set aside time for it.

How much you need to do in order to make a difference might also come as a surprise. As little as half an hour a day will start to enhance your well-being. In guidelines set by governments of the UK, USA and Australia it is suggested that a minimum of just 30 minutes of integrated exercise on five days a week is enough to prevent the risk of obesity and its related problems such as heart disease and diabetes.

So for general health, I recommend trying to incorporate at least half an hour of integrated activity on a daily basis. To get fitter still, or to achieve considerable weight loss, will require a little more effort – around 45–60 minutes daily of integrated activity. But remember, this need not be carried out in a single session – it can be accumulated over the course of a day.

With the integrated exercise plan, the aim is to make activity second nature, so that you barely notice you are doing it; there is no need to do the kind of exercise that leaves you heaving for breath and sweating buckets. Although the more effort you make the sooner you will see results, landmark studies have

strange but true

Juggling balls on a daily basis will increase your calorie burning and boost your brain power. In one study, brainscans of people who had taught themselves to juggle showed that certain areas of the brain had grown.

But beware – whatever you do, don't give up. When the same subjects were tested three months later, during which time they had stopped juggling, their brains had reverted back to their normal size.

confirmed that moderate amounts of activity will keep the pounds off as efficiently as intense exercise sessions.

Researchers found that just half an hour of light activity five days a week was enough for a group of overweight women to slim down and keep the weight off. Those who worked out harder or longer appeared to gain no advantage. The study was the first attempt, by comparing workouts of different durations and intensity, to establish exactly how much exercise is required to stay healthy. The results showed an average 9 per cent weight loss regardless of which programme the women followed, even if they had doubled their daily exercise levels. Tests also showed that the women experienced similar benefits to their hearts and cardiovascular systems.

So, the message is to integrate exercise when and however you can. Your goal is 30 minutes, but beyond that the sky is your limit.

your daily integrated exercise points plan

The points plan on the next few pages groups activities according to their intensity and awards an appropriate number of points to each. You will see, for instance, that you will need to perform a gold-standard activity for less time than a silver- or bronze-standard one to get your points. None of these activities needs to be done in a single burst – 5 minutes of skipping in the morning and 5 in the afternoon is as good for you as 10 minutes at lunchtime. The important thing is to get into the habit of totting up the total time you spend being active within 24 hours.

To improve general health, your daily target should be to amass at least 35 points (or 245 a week). The rate at which you progress your integrated exercise is up to you, but ideally you should aim to accumulate 45–60 points throughout a day (315–420 a week) within four to six months of starting the plan. As long as you don't increase the amount of calories you eat within the average 24 hours (see Chapter 9) and you continue to integrate exercise consistently, you will almost certainly lose weight and maintain that weight loss, as well as see marked improvements in overall health.

However, this plan is designed to be flexible. There will be days on which you are less active than on others, but never lose sight of the fact that the tiniest amount of activity you can muster in a day is better than none. Every step you take (be it up the stairs, walking the dog or pushing a pram) is a step closer to a healthier, happier lifestyle.

work it out

Cracking open **a bottle of wine** in the evening may seem like the perfect way to relax. But you would have to do one of the following to burn off one medium glass of white wine containing 100 calories:

- walk the dog at a steady pace for 16 minutes
- scrub the floor and clean windows vigorously for 22 minutes
- carry heavy bags of groceries for 12.5 minutes
- play tag or rough-and-tumble games with your children for 11 minutes
- wash the car, using plenty of elbow grease and lifting the bucket regularly, for 25 minutes
- repeatedly lift and carry a toddler for 13.5 minutes (you could also try lying on your back and 'bench pressing' a baby for 12 minutes – see page 109)
- get down to some gardening – plenty of raking, hoeing and digging – for 15.5 minutes
- sing and dance along to a CD for 26.5 minutes.

gold-standard integrated activities – perform one of the following for 10 minutes to earn 15 points:

- Brisk walking (a speed of 5mph or faster) that leaves you breathless
- Nordic walking (see page 92)
- Running or jogging at a pace of 10 minutes per mile (or faster)
- Cycling on hilly terrain or at a pace of 10mph or faster
- Continuous skipping
- Continuous leapfrogging
- Continuous piggy backs
- Swimming
- Heavy gardening (digging, carrying heavy loads)
- Mowing the lawn (using a non-motorised lawnmower)
- Shovelling snow
- Moving furniture
- Walking up and down stairs while carrying loads weighing 26kg or more
- Running up and down stairs while carrying a rucksack
- Jogging with your baby in a buggy (see page 112)
- Home repair or construction work – concrete or masonry work, carrying heavy loads up and down a ladder
- Park circuits (see page 114)
- Pogo stick (see page 127)
- Tree-climbing (see page 128)
- Wakeboarding (see page 139)
- Kayaking (see page 139)
- Pushing someone in a wheelchair
- Sawing wood by hand
- Playing any competitive sport
- Rowing

silver-standard integrated activities – perform one of the following for 10 minutes to earn 10 points:

- Cycling on flat ground at a steady pace (5–9mph)
- Walking up and down stairs
- Buggy workouts (see page 111)
- Raking leaves or grass
- Vigorous housework (moving furniture, vacuuming, etc.)
- Painting and decorating
- Cleaning the car
- Walking on sand or stony ground
- Light gardening
- Stripping wallpaper
- Plumbing
- Laying decking
- Putting together flat-pack furniture
- Clearing out a garage or shed
- Sexercise (see page 118)
- Playing with/carrying a toddler
- Walking with a baby in a sling (see page 106)
- Baby-flexing (see page 106)
- Vigorous dancing
- Playing a musical instrument while marching/dancing/walking
- Hopscotch (see page 126)
- Spacehopping (see page 127)
- Carrying shopping bags to the car/home
- Supermarket workout (see page 80)
- Walking on crutches
- Roller skating/inline skating
- Carrying a backpack while shopping
- Riding a pedalo (see page 139)
- Sea-walking (see page 138)
- Building sandcastles (see page 139)
- Golf
- Horse riding
- Playing table tennis
- Line dancing
- Hotel-room workout (see page 140)

bronze-standard integrated activities – perform one of the following for 10 minutes to earn 5 points:

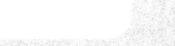

- Car exercises (see page 101)
- Plane/train exercises (see page 136)
- Deskercise (see page 48)
- Fidgeting
- Walking on the spot
- Light housework (dusting, etc.)
- Putting up party decorations/ decorating the Christmas tree
- Sofacise (see page 62)
- Walking the dog
- Washing and drying dishes
- Hanging out the washing
- Ironing
- Dressing/bathing a baby
- Laughing heartily
- Gentle dancing
- Playing a musical instrument
- Putting shopping away
- Hula hooping
- Skating on wheeled trainers
- Jet skiing
- Taking a stroll
- Throwing a frisbee
- Downhill skiing
- Ice skating
- Fishing
- Playing on park/playground equipment
- Playing the drums
- Singing

how fit are you?

Almost everyone is suited to integrated exercise. Because you can select from such a wide range of activities, there will be something within these pages to suit all body types and shapes.

Are you fit to get fit?

Before you become more active there are a number of questions you should ask yourself:

- Do you have a history of heart disease in your close family?
- Do you ever feel pain in your chest muscles when you are active?
- Do you have high blood pressure (i.e. above 160/90)?
- Do you have any old injuries that cause pain when you move?
- Do you suffer from arthritis or osteoporosis?
- Do you suffer from back pain?
- Are you pregnant?
- Do you feel dizzy or faint when you exert yourself?
- Are you in the risky waistband category (see below)?
- Do you have any other health worries that have prevented you from exercising regularly in the past?

If you answered yes to any of the above, it is important to see your GP for a health check before you embark on any form of exercise. In fact, having a medical check-up is wise for anyone who hasn't exercised in a while.

Don't rely on your BMI

For years, working out whether you are too heavy for your size and build has boiled down to using an equation called the Body Mass Index (or BMI). Devised by the nineteenth-century Belgian statistician Adolphe Quetelet, the BMI has been used to define weight for more than a hundred years. Part of its appeal is the simplicity of its calculation: your weight in kilograms is divided by your height in metres squared – the resulting figure being your BMI. A BMI of less than 18.5 is considered 'underweight', between 18.5 and 24.9 is 'normal', 25 to 29.9 is 'overweight' and a BMI of 30 or greater is 'clinically obese'.

The downside of the BMI is that it does not take into account body composition, i.e. whether excess weight is fat or muscle. This is why fit, muscular people often find themselves in the fat or obese categories of the BMI rating system. Many nutrition scientists and health professionals now prefer to use either a waist circumference measurement or a waist-to-height ratio, both of which are considered more accurate indicators of health status.

What is your waist circumference?

A waist circumference measurement is a direct measure of the part of the body that tends to accumulate fat. Using a tape measure positioned around your belly button area, measure around your middle. A measurement of more than 88cm for women and 102cm for men indicates the highest risk of cardio-vascular and metabolic disease (see page 54),

There is still an increased risk of the diseases for women whose measurement is over 80cm and men whose measurement is over 94cm.

Are you an apple or a pear?

Total body fat is not the only indicator of weight-related health problems. The way in which the fat is distributed also plays an important role. For example, body fat that accumulates around the waist, known as abdominal fat (giving you an 'apple' shape) poses a greater health risk than fat that is carried in the hips and thighs (giving you a 'pear' shape). Men are genetically predisposed to gain weight around their waists, although there are exceptions. By contrast, pre-menopausal women's bodies tend to be more 'pear shaped', while post-menopause, a drop in levels of the female hormone oestrogen sees many women gaining weight in a more masculine way – around the middle. Of the two, pear-shapes are healthier. Apple-shaped people have more visceral fat (that which is carried around the internal organs), substantially increasing the risk of heart disease, metabolic syndrome and diabetes.

To work out which shape you are, you need to find your waist-to-hip ratio (WHR). Using a tape measure, if you have a visible waist, measure around the narrowest part; if you don't, measure around the widest part of your middle, usually about 3cm above your navel. That figure is your waist circumference. Next, measure around your hips, just below the point where the top of the thighbone meets the pelvis. Now divide your waist measurement by your hip measurement to get your WHR. If your WHR is 0.80 or lower, your body is a pear shape. If it is higher than 0.80, you are an unhealthier apple shape.

work it out

Mince pies may seem a healthier treat than a chocolate cake at the coffee shop, but do you know how many calories you are nibbling as you munch your way through them? An individual iced fruit pie has around 190 calories, 7g of fat and over 26g (more than five teaspoons) of sugar. A deep-filled pie will deliver a whopping 215 calories, 8g of fat and over 19g of sugar. Add a dollop of cream to the average mince pie and you are looking at 368 calories and 25g of fat. To get that off you would need to do one of the following:

- stand up and sit down repetitively for 90 minutes
- play the air guitar for 1 hour and 45 minutes
- skip non-stop for 50 minutes
- carry a fairly heavy backpack around with you for 1 hour
- referee (or play in) a kids' football match for 1 hour and 10 minutes
- juggle balls for 95 minutes.

how to measure your fitness levels

It is not strictly necessary to test physiological parameters in order to start this exercise plan. But assessing your current fitness level and retesting yourself every three to four months can be fun, as well as a great way to boost motivation when you see how effective your integrated activity has been. If the results of your tests begin to plateau, it may be time to think about increasing the duration, intensity or frequency of your activity. Here are some simple assessments to help you gauge your progress.

Aerobic fitness

You will need a bench or a low, sturdy chair about 22–25cm high. Keeping your back straight and abdominal muscles tucked in, begin stepping on and off. Keep upright and don't lean forward. Maintain a steady pace for 2 minutes, aiming to take around forty steps a minute. Sit down for half a minute and then take your pulse at your wrist or neck for 15 seconds. Multiply the figure by four to obtain your pulse rate per minute.

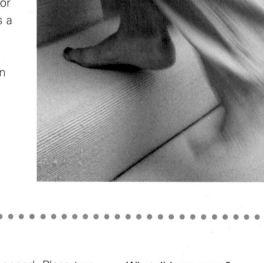

What did you score?
- 92 or less (excellent)
- 92–110 (good)
- 112 plus (average)

Agility

This is how fast you can change direction at speed. Place two 40cm lengths of tape on the floor about 40cm apart. Stand with your right foot on one of the markers and your left foot off the ground. Hop from line to line on your right foot as many times as you can in 15 seconds, subtracting any times you miss the marker. Repeat on your left foot. Add the scores together and divide by two to get an average.

What did you score?
- 26 or more (excellent)
- 21–26 (good)
- 20 or less (average)

Upper-body strength

A good guide to this is how many press-ups you can do in a minute. Make sure you get the technique right: lie on your stomach with your hands beneath your shoulders and your palms flat on the floor. Push your body up to straighten your arms, keeping your lower back straight. Then lower your body to the floor by bending your elbows until your chest is about 30–38cm off the floor.

How many can you do in a minute?
- 25 or more full press ups (excellent)
- 15–24 (good)
- Below 15 (average)

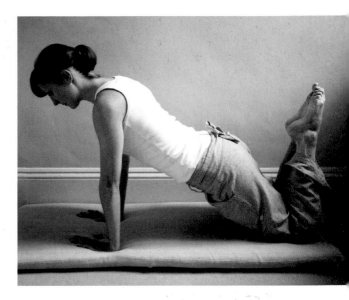

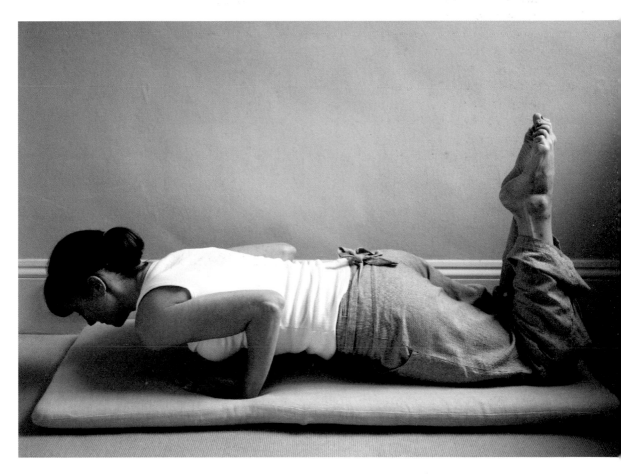

Lower-body flexibility

This tests how flexible you are in your hamstring muscles at the backs of your legs and in your lower back. Sit on the floor, legs together and directly out in front of you. Your bottom and back should be against a door or wall. Slowly lean towards your toes without straining your neck.

How far could you reach with your fingertips?
* To your ankles or beyond (excellent)
* Between knees and ankles (good)
* To your knees (average)

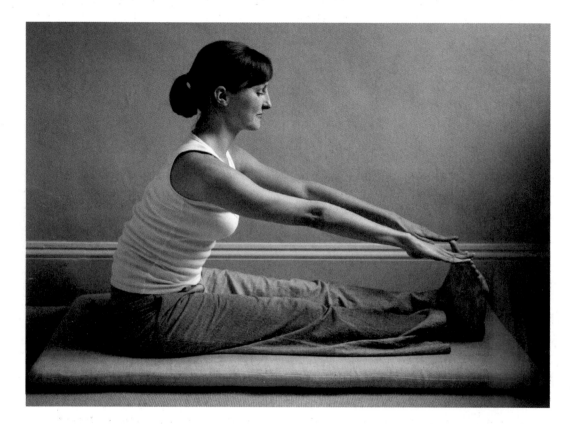

Lower-body strength

Stand with your back against a wall and move your body down and your feet out until your knees are bent at right angles to the floor. Place your hands lightly on your thighs as if you are sitting on a chair, keeping your lower back pressed into the wall.

How long can you manage?
* 3 minutes or more (excellent)
* 90 seconds–3 minutes (good)
* Under 90 seconds (average)

what to wear

Integrated exercise requires no financial outlay and that includes money spent on expensive fitness gear and clothing. Generally, you can get by wearing loose-fitting clothing made from natural fibres (such as cotton) and a comfortable pair of walking shoes or trainers. However, the more activity you do, the more likely it is that you will want to equip yourself with items of clothing made specifically for comfort, breathability and support when you are moving about.

Dress for success

Here is a guide to investing your money wisely should you choose to extend your fitness wardrobe:

Try before you buy. Make sure you try everything on before buying and, if possible, stretch or at least walk around to check that the clothing allows full range of movement and doesn't ride up and down. Look for covered seams that will not chafe your skin.

If most of your exercise will be performed indoors, choose stretchy fabrics that contain a percentage of the elastic fabric Lycra.

The golden rule for outdoor exercise is to layer. Several lightweight base layers keep you warmer than a heavyweight sweatshirt as air will be trapped between the garments. You can also peel off one piece of clothing at a time as you warm up. For outdoor activity a lightweight, breathable jacket is also recommended.

Look for sweat-wicking sports fabrics, such as Nike's Dri-Fit, designed to keep moisture wicked away. They are more expensive than conventional fabrics but they are comfortable and wash well, so are worth the higher financial outlay. Cotton is great, but tends to soak up sweat and moisture causing the skin to become clammy and cold if it is worn for any length of time.

For some activities it is wise to visit a specialist shop for advice. For running or walking, for example, you will need a loose-fitting pair of jogging bottoms or Lycra tights, a T-shirt and some seam-free socks to reduce the risk of blisters. A good pair of running or walking shoes is also essential (see overleaf). Cyclists should invest in a helmet that meets safety standards, a water bottle, puncture repair kit and some padded shorts. If you intend cycling, walking or running in the dark, make sure you invest in reflective strips so that you can be spotted by passing motorists.

Whether or not you have a large bust, all women need to wear a sports bra if they are to perform power-walking, running or other activities that involve a lot of movement. Repetitive and high-impact activity with an inadequate bra means the breasts bounce, stretching their fragile support system to its limits. Over time, this could lead to droopy, sagging breasts and back or shoulder pain. Make sure you get yourself properly fitted – around 85 per cent of women wear the wrong size bra.

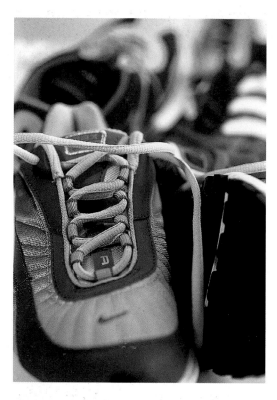

The lowdown on trainers

If you are going to fork out on just one item of clothing for exercise, make it a pair of trainers. Often people make do with old and ill-fitting ones and these can cause anything from a niggle to acute pain or long-term damage to muscles and joints. Trainers have a shelf life of six months to one year, depending on how often you use them and for which activity. But there is no need to spend a fortune on a new pair. Studies by podiatrists have shown that middle-of-the-range trainers are the best buy. Staff at a specialist sports shop will be able to advise you on the correct shoe for you and your chosen activity. Here are some more tips:

Check that there is some tread left on the bottom of your current trainers. If the pattern has worn away completely, invest in a new pair as protection will be reduced.

Most reasonable-quality trainers will have removable insoles. Check them regularly to see if they are worn away at the ball of the foot or the heel – another sign that your shoes have had their day.

Take your old trainers with you to a specialist running shop when you buy a new pair. Staff can tell a lot about the way you run or walk from looking at them.

Always try on new trainers in the afternoon when your feet have swollen and, since feet swell further when you exercise, wear a fairly thick pair of socks to find the best fit.

A common mistake is to buy trainers that are too small which will constrict the toes and increase the risk of bruising on the toenails and heels. In general you will need half a size bigger in sports shoes than in regular footwear. Ideally, your heel should fit snugly in the cup and the fit should be just tight enough to prevent any movement up and down or from side to side when you walk.

Do you need functional footwear?

In the last couple of years, a functional-footwear phenomenon has spurned a hugely competitive market for sandals and trainers that promise more than just comfort and style. If you want to lose weight, tone up flabby parts or just feel healthier, claim the manufacturers of these products, you need do nothing more than change your shoes. Do they work? Some have scientific evidence to support their claims, others are mere marketing hype. But if you like the idea of burning a few extra calories with no extra effort, then Flitflops, Crocs and MBTs are just some of the brands you might consider.

useful tools

If you are tempted to invest in fitness gadgets, think twice before you part with your money. In a study by researchers at Kansas State University, devices that promised a flat stomach with regular use were found wanting. A group of twenty-three men and women used various gadgets – including an abdominal 'roller' and an abdominal 'slider' – while electrodes measured the stimulation to their abdominal muscles. On average, the products elicited no greater muscle activity than would traditional sit-ups.

So instead of investing a small fortune in something that might not even be helpful try substituting ordinary household objects for gym equipment. Here are some suggestions for 'gadgets' that you probably already have in your home, but feel free to use your initiative and imagination to come up with more:

Home equipment

- **Plastic bottles** filled with sand or water make ideal hand weights. Vary the size for lighter and heavier weights.
- **A garden bench** is great for performing step-ups.
- **A dining chair** can also be used for 'sofacise' (see page 62).
- **Tinned foods** make ideal, lighter hand weights.
- **A length of washing line** makes an instant skipping rope.
- **Crowbars and sledgehammers** can be used as weight-training tools.
- **Stairs** are the perfect alternative to the gym's stairclimber.
- **Lawnmowers and vacuum cleaners** are great for resistance training.

chapter two

We are, notoriously, a generation of workaholics. Statistics show that most people in Europe work at least 48 hours a week; in some countries, such as the UK, as many as one in twenty-five people works a 60-hour week or longer. The amount of time we spend at our desk or workplace could be seriously damaging our health, as well as making us stressed and, in some cases, miserable, inactive and prone to piling on the pounds.

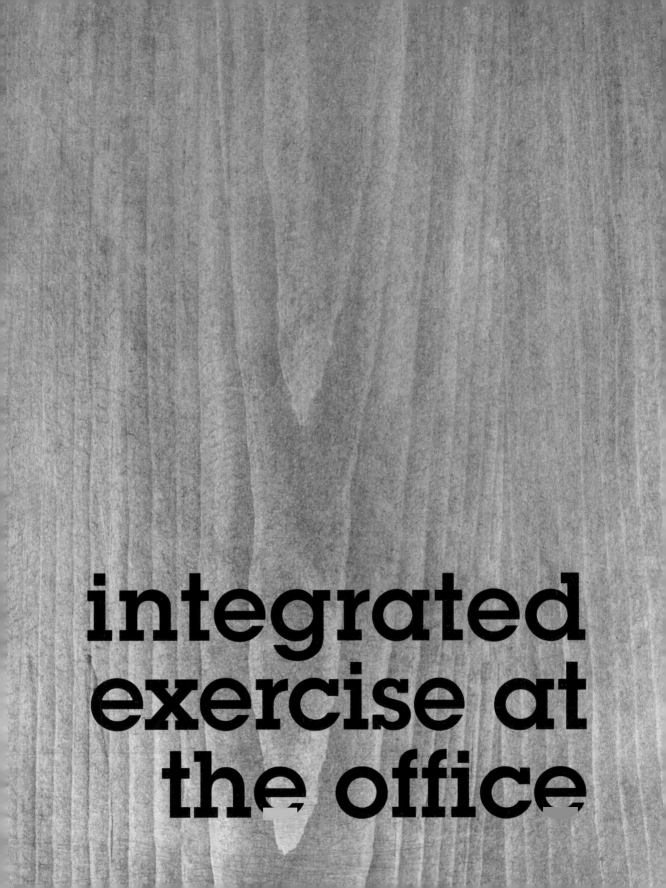

integrated exercise at the office

are you a desk potato?

An Australian study suggested the workplace is increasingly to blame for the obesity epidemic: the longer people sit at their desks, the more likely they are to be overweight. Workers sat an average of more than 3 hours a day, with 25 per cent sedentary for more than 6 hours a day. Men sat an average of 209 minutes on the job (20 minutes more than women). That extra 20 minutes men spend off their feet appeared to make a difference with their inactivity leading to a higher incidence of obesity.

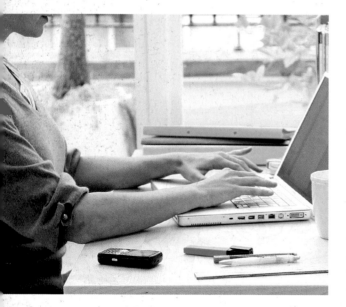

Sedentary office-based workers, dubbed 'desk potatoes', spend so many hours sitting at their desk that they are at risk of deep vein thrombosis (DVT), a condition which causes potentially fatal blood clots that can travel to the heart, lungs or brain. DVT is most commonly associated with passengers on long-haul flights without space to move in cramped seats. But of sixty-two people presenting at hospitals in New Zealand with blood clots, 34 per cent had been sitting at their desks for long periods. Many were going 3–4 hours at a time without getting up and those most at risk of DVT sat in front of their screens for a staggering 14 hours a day.

Of course, DVT is not the only health threat. Expanding waistlines are literally weighing workers down with many people finding their burgeoning weight affecting their mental output as well as their physical health.

And if you need even more incentive to get moving, consider the fact that it might improve your job prospects. A survey of employers showed that they thought obesity affected productivity and also that they believed overweight people lacked self-discipline.

The fact is that there really is no excuse not to get more active even if you are at your desk most of the day. And the best news of all is that there are lots of easy ways to do it that don't involve losing your lunch hour to the gym.

twelve great ways to integrate exercise into your working day

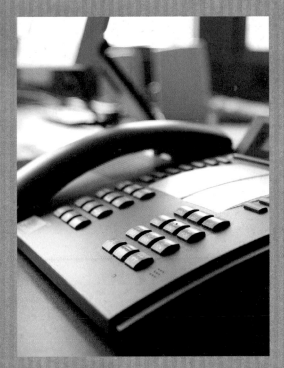

1 Set your alarm 30 minutes earlier and walk to the station or to the shops to get a paper or cycle to work.

2 If you drive to work, park at the farthest end of the car park.

3 Practise deskercise exercises (see page 48) as often as you can – at least a couple an hour.

4 Walk to deliver messages to colleagues in the same building whenever you can.

5 Use the stairs instead of the lift or escalator.

6 Use the toilets furthest from your desk.

7 Stand up when you are talking on the phone.

8 Suggest a walking meeting to your colleagues – the fresh air may trigger more creative thoughts and the walking will get you fitter.

9 Send printing jobs to the printer farthest from your desk.

10 Walk to buy your lunch or eat your lunch in a park and go for a walk afterwards.

11 Try an 'e-mail-free Friday' – the idea being for employers to ban all internal e-mails every Friday in order to get employees walking around the office more.

12 Ask your employer if they run any schemes to encourage activity among workers such as providing showers in the office for active employees who want to run or cycle to work (or at lunchtime) or bike-loan facilities.

deskercise

Research has shown that millions of hours of vital exercise are being lost due to the explosion of e-mail. Whereas staff were once forced to walk to their colleagues' desks to pass on information, the e-mail revolution now means much of this can be done with a tap of the computer keyboard. Almost half of workers admitted in one survey to e-mailing the person sitting next to them to avoid making verbal contact.

When walking is not possible these desk exercises are the next best thing. Ideally, perform at least two desk exercises every hour – anything is better than sitting in the same position – and remember to breathe normally while holding your body in one of the stretching positions.

Hamstring hug

This exercise stretches the hamstring muscles in the backs of the legs which become tight after sitting down for too long.

1 Sit back in your chair and place your hands under your right thigh.

2 Pull your knee towards your chest then extend the leg straight in front of you as far as you can. Relax and repeat with the other leg.

Repeat 3–5 times with each leg.

Pelvic tilt

This exercise involves only a very small movement, but is effective at toning the pelvic-floor muscles that are also crucial for maintaining abdominal strength.

Sit tall on your chair. Tighten your abdominal muscles and bring the pubic bone upwards.

Repeat 20 times.

Vertical stretches

This is the perfect way to relieve stress and tension throughout the body.

1 Stand up with your feet shoulder-width apart. Raise up on your toes, extending your arms overhead.

2 Reach as high as possible with each hand alternately for 5 seconds.

Relax, and repeat 5 times on each side.

Head tilt

Neck muscles get tight from sitting at your computer and from cradling the phone in your neck. Here's a simple exercise to remedy this.

Slowly bend your head to the right as far as possible, then to the left, then forwards (your chin against your throat) and backwards.

Repeat twice in each direction.

Self-hug

This exercise stretches out the muscles in the back and shoulders.

Bring your arms across your chest, trying to reach as far around the back as possible. Hold for 10 seconds.

Relax and repeat with the other arm on top.

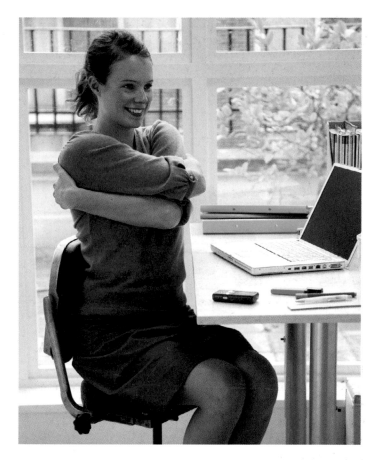

Foot exercises

Simple moves such as rotating the ankles and wiggling the toes prevents the blood from pooling in the feet and then struggling to climb up through the veins, the principal causes of DVT.

Chest stretch

Problems can arise when weak chest muscles (or pectorals) become tight and shortened as a result of being hunched over a desk (or steering wheel) for hours on end. This exercise will help by stretching these muscles.

1 Sit with your feet hip-width apart, your elbows tucked in at the waist, palms on your knees and facing upwards. Breathe in and sit up straight, keeping your neck relaxed. Breathe out, slowly.

2 Breathe in again and, keeping elbows at your waist, draw your forearms sidewards to open out the chest. Do not let your shoulders rise up. Breathe out.

Repeat 5 times.

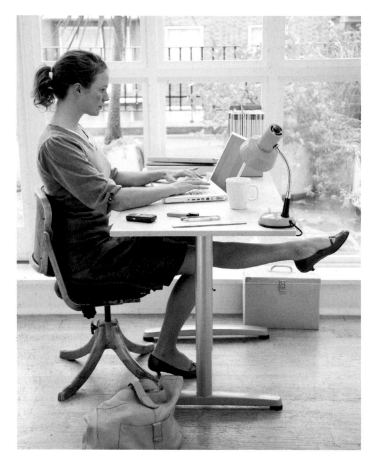

Leg extensions

This is a good exercise to strengthen your legs and it can be done under your desk so nobody notices.

1 Raise one foot about 2.5cm off the ground.

2 Bring the foot upwards and forwards (your toes should be aligned with your knee), then lower it back down without allowing it to touch the floor.

Repeat 12 times before changing sides.

Phone muscle stretch

Half of office workers who use a telephone for at least 2 hours a day and also use a computer report neck pain according to the UK-based charity Back Care. Cradling a phone can cause compression of the vertebrae in the neck and tight muscles in the shoulders. Over time that can lead to muscular and postural imbalances in the neck, shoulders and upper back. In the long term, consistently bad phone posture can cause wear and tear to the shoulder joints resulting in osteoarthritic changes such as small calcium deposits forming on tendons. Stretching after a phone call can really help.

1 Tuck in your chin, bend your right ear towards your right shoulder and allow the left shoulder to drop.

2 Place your right hand on the left side of your head and pull your head very gently. (Keep your eyes down – if you look up you will strain your neck muscles.) Hold for 30 seconds.

Repeat on the other side to un-kink muscles thoroughly.

Wrist flexion and hyperextension

One in fifty people suffers from repetitive strain injury (RSI) resulting in 5.4 million working days being lost each year. A painful condition that creeps up on sufferers, it is caused by a swelling of the tissue in or near the narrow passageway of the wrist, called the carpal tunnel. This swelling puts pressure on the median nerve, leading to the symptoms of pain, tingling, weakness or numbness that are associated with RSI.

1 For wrist flexion, gently apply force with your left hand to stretch your right wrist towards the underside of the right forearm. Hold for 3–5 seconds, then relax and repeat with the other side.

Repeat 5 times with each wrist.

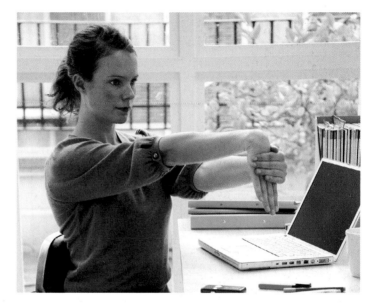

2 For wrist hyperextension, gently apply force with your left palm to bend your right hand backwards. Hold for 3–5 seconds, then relax and repeat with the other side.

Repeat 5 times with each wrist.

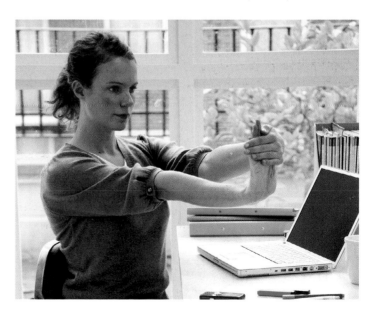

Side bends

This exercise helps to strengthen and stretch the abdominal muscles.

1 Sit on a chair, feet flat on the floor, hands at your sides.

2 Bend over as far as is comfortable, hands reaching towards or touching the floor. Hold for 3–5 seconds, then slowly pull your body back up into a sitting position while tightening your abdominal muscles.

Relax and repeat 5 times on each side.

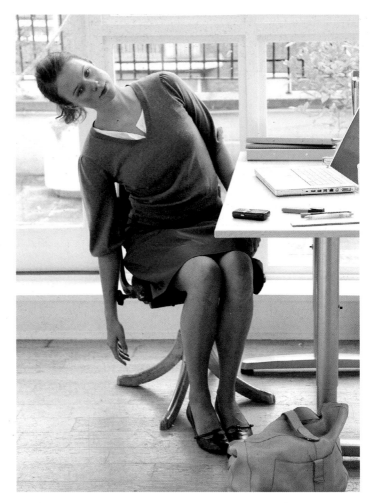

And finally, some heavy breathing

Here's an exercise to relax you whenever you feel tired or tense. All you need is a quiet spot where you can sit down.

1 Close your eyes and breathe in deeply through your nose to the count of 5.

2 Exhale to the count of 5 through your mouth. Shut out the noise and distractions around you by concentrating on the air flowing in and out of your body.

Keep breathing deeply like this for at least 5 minutes.

futuristic office fitness

If the majority of your day is spent sitting in front of a computer screen, you might think it is impossible to burn calories while you work. But in the office of the future, things might be very different. Instead of sitting at your desk, you would work standing up. And instead of standing still, you would be walking on a treadmill. Meetings might be conducted while walking laps of a simulated athletics track.

This might sound too sci-fi to be true, but researchers at the Mayo Clinic showed that not only is it possible to perform routine office work while walking very slowly on a treadmill built into a workstation, but that about 120 extra calories an hour can be burned while doing so. A specially designed vertical workstation allowed workers to operate a standard personal computer while walking on an integrated treadmill at a pace of 1 mile per hour.

True multi-tasking

Designed by Professor James Levine and his colleagues at the Mayo, the workstation is supported by four locking rubber wheels so that it can be moved around easily. As well as housing a computer, keyboard and mouse, it even incorporates an area to hold flowers, pens and a coffee cup. In the study, subjects were able to take telephone calls, check their e-mails or continue typing as they walked. Levine, who led the study, suggested that using the treadmill on just three working days

a week could achieve a weight loss of almost a kilogram a month.

It might not be long before forward-thinking companies invest in equipment such as this. In the meantime, remember to stand up when you are talking on the phone, and to walk around the office as often as you can.

work it out

If you think your pre-work **coffee** habit is calorie-kind, then you are very much mistaken. That cappuccino you grab on the way to work probably contains 180 calories and 9g of fat. And if it's a caramel cappuccino you can almost double the calorie count. So to work off those 180 calories you would need to do one of the following:

- push a pram or buggy (with a baby or toddler in it) for 40 minutes
- walk up and down stairs, fully clothed, for 35 minutes
- rake up autumn leaves for 45 minutes
- walk to a supermarket or shop 15 minutes away and walk back carrying bags
- dance fairly vigorously for 35 minutes
- play tag with your children for 40 minutes
- sit writing at your desk for 1 hour and 40 minutes.

exercise the stress away

Stress at work is unhealthy in many ways, not least in that it can make you fat. American scientists looked at the way sixty women reacted to levels of stress in their lives and found that the more tension they had to deal with, the more fatty baggage they accumulated around their abdomens. Experts believe that raised levels of cortisol, the hormone produced by stress, are responsible for this. The theory is that higher levels of circulating stress hormones affect the type of fat that settles beneath the abdominal wall.

This is perhaps one reason why people who suffer from chronic stress caused by their job are more likely to develop heart disease and diabetes. One British study looked at the stress levels reported by more than 10,000 civil servants, aged 35 to 55, in twenty government departments. Researchers found that those who most often reported stress were most likely to have a set of risk factors for heart disease and diabetes, which included abdominal obesity, raised cholesterol and high blood pressure, known collectively as metabolic syndrome.

And the best way to combat stress? Get moving. In the UK, the Mental Health Foundation urges GPs to offer exercise on prescription to people suffering from stress and the mild to moderate depression it sometimes causes. One study found that levels of the chemical phenylethylamine (similar in structure to amphetamines) increase substantially during a workout to produce a significant mood-boosting effect.

As we've already seen, any sort of activity can help. Often, the mere fact that you are doing something positive rather than sitting behind your desk will raise your mood, but exercise can also get rid of physical and mental tension. The amount needed to achieve these effects varies, but psychologists have found that many people feel better after just a few minutes of activity such as a brisk walk if they do it regularly. Researchers found that the benefits of a daily 20-minute walk were comparable to improvements gained on a stress-management course.

It pays to take an exercise break

So whenever you feel you are drowning at work, the key may be not to take a lunch or coffee break, but simply to get moving. Research has proven that busy professionals who exercise during the day feel more productive. They're also less likely to spout off at colleagues or slam down the phone after they've worked up a sweat.

In a study of about 200 workers at three sites (a university, a computer company and a life-insurance firm), employees were asked to complete questionnaires about their job performance and mood on days when they exercised at work and days when they didn't. Free to take part in any physical activity – from a stroll to yoga – most participants spent 30–60 minutes during their lunch hour doing some type of physical activity.

Six out of ten workers said their time-management skills, mental performance and ability to meet deadlines improved on days when they exercised, the overall performance boost being about 15 per cent. Crucially, neither the type of activity nor its duration seemed to make a difference. All that mattered was that they were active.

did you know?

Slouching at your desk is a real no-no for maintaining good posture and strong core muscles, but some office chairs give you a workout as you work.

- A saddle seat (such as those made by Bambach (see page 160) is a great example. Ergonomically designed to allow your spine to function within its optimal, natural curve it strengthens core stability muscles while relaxing those in the shoulders. Researchers found that subjects performed significantly better in upper-limb tasks when sitting on a saddle seat as opposed to a normal one.

- Sitting on a Swiss Ball also has positive effects — the instability of the ball means your abdominal muscles must work hard just to keep you upright.
  However, physiotherapists recommend easing yourself into using these means of sitting as your core muscles need to be strong to use them appropriately.

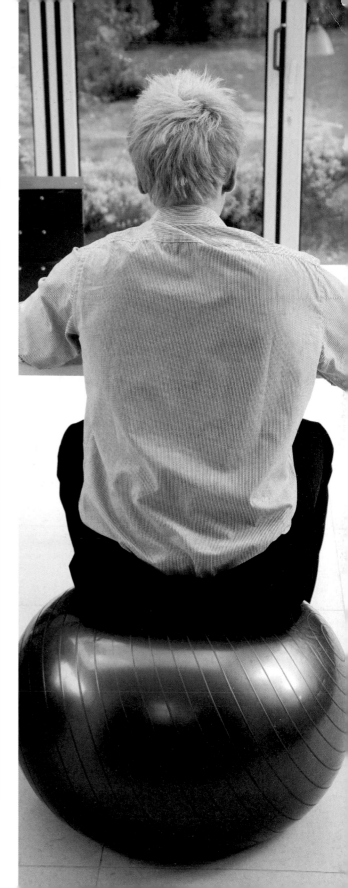

chapter three

The worst thing about spending much of your time at home is that household chores seem never-ending. Just as you finish gardening, the car needs cleaning or the dog needs walking and so on. But this treadmill of domesticity can provide the workout equivalent of cross-training. Every muscle in the body will be used and many of the tasks will also work your heart and lungs. In fact, the best place to begin integrating exercise is at home.

integrated exercise at home

housework-out

Even in these days of cleaners as well as labour-saving vacuums, dishwashers and washing machines, surveys show that the average woman (and some men) spends 12.8 hours a week cleaning her home. Sounds like bad news until you consider that dusting, vacuuming and scrubbing are, according to several studies, as effective for losing that flab as pumping iron at the gym.

For instance, research in Germany found that around 35–40 minutes spent cleaning windows burns 250 calories, washing the car burns 330 and ironing a load of laundry 210. This compares favourably with activities that you might perform in the gym, such as cycling on an exercise bike for 10 minutes, which burns 50–60 calories.

Household chores offer considerable disease-fighting benefits too. A study of some 413,000 people in ten European countries suggested that those who regularly did housework were less likely to develop cancer of the colon. Other studies have shown that daily housework cut the risk of endometrial cancer by 30 per cent and increased the chance of women surviving breast cancer. And in Australian research, simple household tasks such as doing the laundry, ironing or washing-up were found to reduce the risk of diabetes and heart disease. High glucose levels are associated with diabetes and cardiovascular disease and the scientists found that doing chores was beneficially associated with lower blood glucose levels.

did you know?

If you suffer from back pain, there are a few tips that can make housework less aggravating.

- Don't bend over when cleaning the bath, dusting the skirting boards or reaching low shelves: squat or kneel instead.

- An upright vacuum cleaner is best for your back. Keep it close to your body, using short sweeping movements backwards and forwards.

- Ensure that you have easy access to each side of your bed so you don't have to stretch when making it and kneel or squat to tuck in sheets and blankets.

- Rest every so often when doing a long job. Change position and stretch, or change tasks.

Polishing

If you need to dust a lot of high shelves or move trinkets, the benefits of this chore are great. Much of the work is done when you stretch as you reach out with your duster – you will be working your arms, the pectoral muscles in your chest and your shoulders. Polishing brass items or shoes usually involves a scrubbing motion and this works muscles in the forearms, biceps and triceps. Move the brush or pad quickly and swap hands to avoid muscular imbalance.

As you polish, try some buttock clenching (see page 136). On the last count, squeeze the gluteal muscles hard before relaxing – this will help to keep your bottom pert.

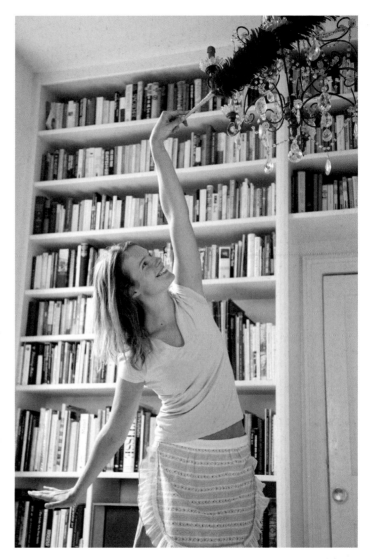

Washing and ironing

When you are loading the washing machine, remember to squat rather than bend from the waist – it will work your thigh and buttock muscles. Hanging out the clothes to dry will tax your arms and shoulders and ironing them afterwards is best for the upper body. Remember to alternate the iron between your hands if you can so that your preferred hand does not do all the work, and make sure that the board is not positioned too low or too high, which will strain and stress your back.

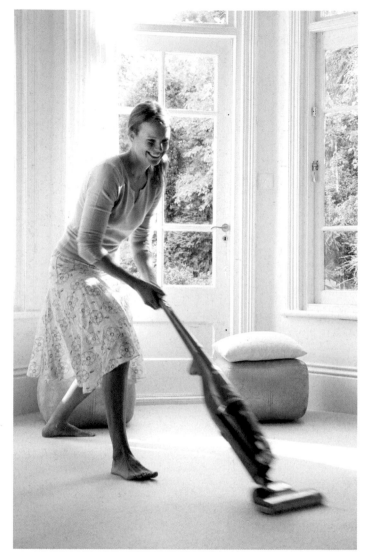

Vacuuming

This is a good form of resistance training. Before you start, try doing some squats if you have an upright vacuum cleaner:

1 Stand back from the vac with your feet hip-width apart and your back straight, supporting yourself by placing your hands on the handle of the machine.

2 Bend your knees and, keeping your back straight, stick your bottom out so that you can feel your legs working as you lower towards the floor. Hold for a couple of seconds then return to the start position.

Repeat 10–15 times.

When you start vacuuming, work the muscles in your arms by pushing and pulling vigorously with the machine. As you push you use the biceps muscles in the front of your arms as well as chest and shoulder muscles. When you pull, you work the triceps muscles at the back of your arms. To work up a sweat, try to do the entire house in one go rather than taking a breather between rooms. And try changing the settings so that the brush is at its greatest resistance – making it harder to push and pull will give you a better workout.

Cleaning the car

It might take longer than a garage car wash, but the bucket-and-sponge approach to cleaning your vehicle is well worth it when it comes to calorie burning. Scrubbing the wheels and paintwork will work your arms and abdominal muscles, as will vacuuming and wiping the interior. Throwing buckets of water to rinse away the soapy suds is all good strength training. Using a hosepipe lessens the strengthening benefits, but is a workout all the same.

Mopping

Before you start, try some lunges using the mop for support. When the American Council on Exercise commissioned a study to find the best bottom exercises, they found that lunges were among the most effective for targeting the leg and gluteal muscles together:

1 Hold the mop so that the head is on the floor in front of you at right angles to the floor.

2 Hold with both hands and step forwards into a lunge position – your right knee should be above your right heel and your left leg bent at the knee behind you. Lower your hips and left knee towards the floor.

Hold for 5 seconds and return to the start position before repeating on the other side.

When you mop, use lots of elbow grease. Holding in your stomach muscles (but remembering to breathe!) as you work. Lift the bucket with both hands so that you don't overwork one side of the body.

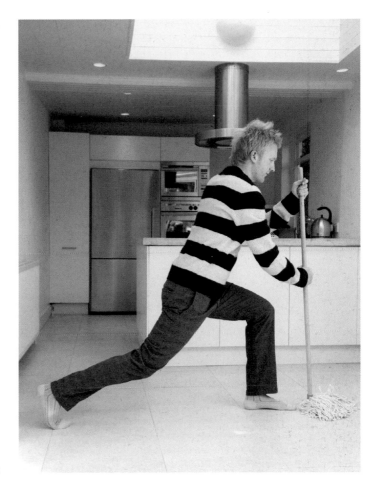

Washing windows

Obviously, the size and position of your windows has a big part to play in the effectiveness of this chore. If they are very high or large and require you to climb on and off a chair or ladder to reach them, all the better in terms of your housework-out. Make it harder still by stretching upwards higher than usual to work your back and shoulder muscles. Avoid any twisting movements of the spine, which can strain the lower back, and don't stretch to the point of discomfort. If you find it difficult, move a little closer to the window so that the large muscle groups do more work. If you are using a bucket, don't put it right next to you – leave it where you need to reach for it, remembering to bend your knees as you do so.

sofacise

Slump into your sofa and reach for the remote control if you will, but the latest research suggests that if you do so too often square eyes will be the least of your worries. According to some surveys, we have become such a generation of couch potatoes that we now spend an average of 14 years of our lives snuggled up between cushions in front of the box.

And it is not just our waistlines that suffer as a consequence of our sofa habits. Scientists from the World Health Organisation (WHO) have stated that our couch-potato way of life is more damaging to health than smoking. Whereas smoking causes 9 per cent of all chronic diseases in Europe, physical inactivity and poor diet combined were found to be responsible for 10 per cent. Other research carried out by physiotherapists showed that sitting with the spine in a C position (as most people do on a sofa) rather than with an S-shaped spine increases the risk of back problems in later life.

But fear not, because your humble sofa or armchair can soon be transformed into a workout station. And here's how.

Before you start

Much of the sofacise workout can be done on your sofa or armchair, but for some optional exercises you will need a sturdier dining chair. Remember that you should always move in a controlled and smooth manner – if you are jerking or straining your limbs and muscles then you are trying too hard and your efforts will be counterproductive.

For added resistance some of the moves can be performed using two tins of baked beans, two bottles of water or even a pair of socks filled with coins and secured at the ends – all work well as alternatives to the kind of hand weights used in gyms.

Start each exercise by sitting with the backs of your thighs supported by the chair or sofa and feet flat on the floor. Your back should be straight, so lengthen your spine and sit tall, pulling your tummy muscles in. Relax your shoulders, keep your head straight and allow your arms to hang down by your sides between exercises.

Warm up

Do at least 5 minutes stretching before you start. Sit on the floor and reach backwards, forwards and to the sides with your hands. Then, sitting on the sofa or armchair, do these warm-up moves:

Arm swing

Swing your arms forwards and upwards in a wide arc 4 times.

Shake it out

Flick your fingers and hands downwards 8 times in front of your body, 8 times overhead and 8 times with your hands hanging at your sides. Tap your toes and heels at the same time.

Head turn

Turn your head slowly and carefully to the right, then to the front, then the left.

Repeat 4 times.

Shoulder roll

Roll your shoulders forwards 4 times and backwards 4 times while maintaining a good upright position.

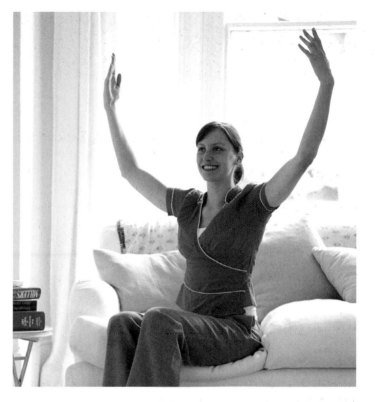

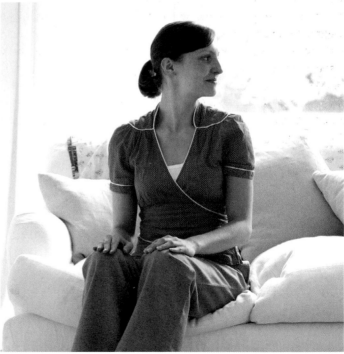

Chest press

1 Hold a filled water bottle or can in each hand and bend your arms so that your upper arms are parallel to the floor and out to the sides of your body. Keep your elbows at shoulder height.

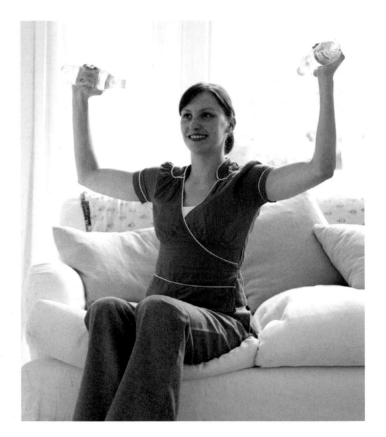

Sofa dips

It is best to do these exercises using the outside arm of the sofa because you need a firm surface.

1 Sit on the sofa arm and place both hands on the edge, one each side of your bottom. Your knees should be hip-width apart and your thighs at right angles to the floor, although you can make the move more challenging by moving your feet further away from your body.

2 Shuffle your bottom off the sofa by supporting your weight with your arms. Bend your arms and lower your body. Keep your back straight and as close to the sofa as possible, and your lower abdominal muscles tight. Lower your body until your upper arms are parallel to the floor. Straighten your arms slowly.

Repeat 15 times.

2 Slowly move your arms towards your front until your hands meet together at the front of your face.

Repeat 12–15 times.

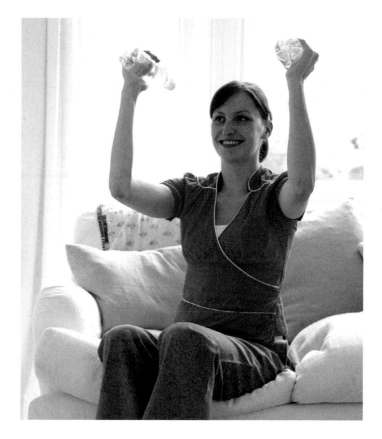

Triceps scissors

1 Holding the cans behind you with arms almost straight (so that your palms are facing backwards), squeeze your shoulder blades together.

2 With your arms as straight as possible, try to reach or push upwards with your hands behind your back so that your right and left hands are alternately on top in a scissor-like movement.

Repeat 12–15 times.

Biceps curl

1 Keeping your elbows into the sides of your waist, hold a tin of beans in each hand with thumbs facing outwards.

2 Raise your hands slowly towards your shoulders and lower back down to the starting position.

Repeat 12–15 times.

Overhead press

1 Holding a can in each hand, bend your arms so that your hands are almost level with your shoulders.

2 Slowly push towards the ceiling and return to the starting position.

Repeat 12–15 times.

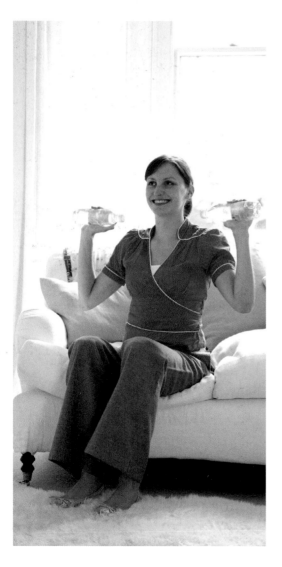

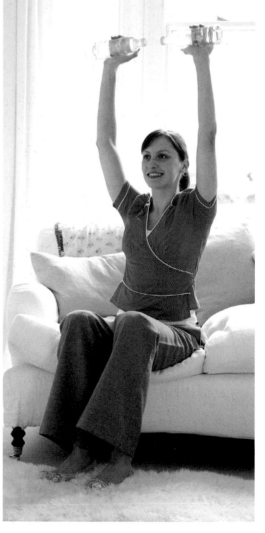

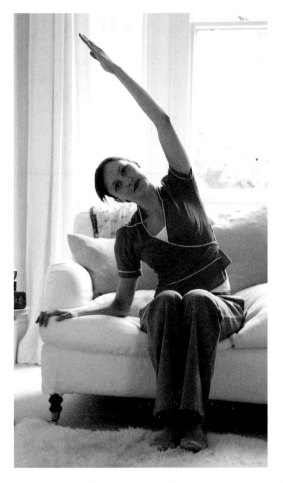

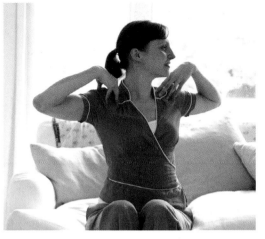

Side twists

1 Keep your buttocks on the seat and place your hands on your shoulders.

2 Raise your elbows to the side at shoulder height (or lower if you find this difficult). Keep your elbows raised and gently twist your shoulders alternately to the right, then to the front, then to the left.

Repeat 12–15 times.

Side bends

1 Keeping both buttocks on the seat, imagine you are in between panes of double glazing and can move neither forwards nor backwards.

2 Bend to the right for 4 counts, hold in position for 4 counts and come up again in 4 counts.

Repeat 12 times on each side.

Pelvic tilt

This is a very small but very effective movement for toning the lower-stomach area.

Sit tall and pull your tummy button back to your spine. Tighten your lower abdominal muscles and bring the pubic bone forwards and upwards.

Repeat 12–15 times.

Single-leg squat

Research has proven this is the best exercise for toning the buttocks.

Sit on the edge of the seat. Stand up on one leg (keeping your knee flexed and holding your arms out for balance) and then slowly return to the seated position.

Repeat 12 times on each leg.

TIP: If you find this too difficult, practise two-legged squats until you gain sufficient leg-strength to try the one-legged variety.

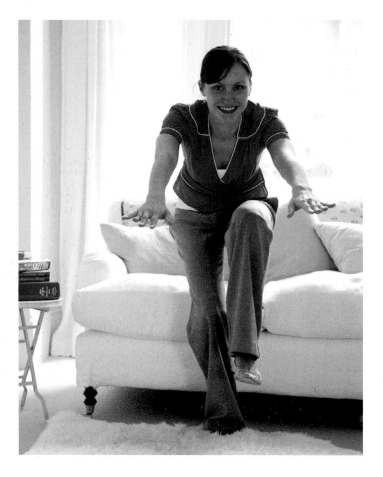

Buttock squeeze

Sit tall with your feet flat on the floor. Squeeze your buttocks together tightly and release.

Repeat 20 times.

Leg extensions

1 Sitting upright, with your bottom towards the edge of the sofa, place your hands on either side of your body holding the edge for support and raise one foot about 2.5cm off the ground.

2 Bring the foot and straightened leg upwards (toes should be aligned with the knee) and then down without allowing the foot to touch the floor for 12 repetitions.

Repeat with the other leg.

Knee lifts

Sitting tall, lift and lower one bent knee 15 times without allowing your foot to touch the floor until the final repetition.

Repeat with the other knee.

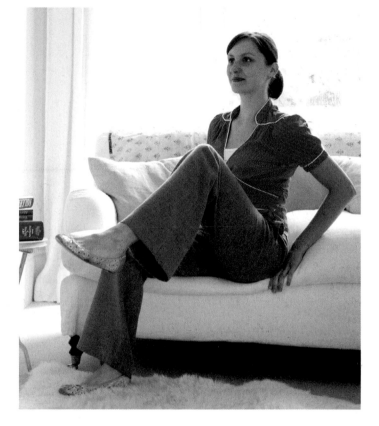

Channel-hopping lunges

Make sure you put some effort into switching channels by getting into this habit every time you want to watch a different programme.

1 Stand up and put your right foot one large stride in front of your left, keeping you're hips square to the front.

2 Once you've changed channel, allow your arms to hang loosely by your sides.

3 Bend your knees so that you bring your right knee directly over your right foot, and lower your body, taking about three seconds to do so. Keep your weight on the heel of your front foot so that you really work your buttock muscles.

Raise yourself back to the start position and repeat 10 times.

dog walking

If there is one way to ensure that you integrate exercise into your daily life, it is to get a dog. My dog – Bobo, a border collie – is not only a great companion, but a walking, woofing, four-legged alternative to a gym membership. And countless studies have shown that dog owners lead healthier lives with lower blood pressure and cholesterol and fewer minor ailments and serious medical problems.

Taking over the family dog-walking duties will benefit both you and your pooch. Walking the dog for just 20 minutes a day, five days a week, produced an average weight loss of over 6kg for participants in one study.

Other research has shown how walking the dog can also ward off depression and loneliness. Dogs help to motivate their owners by encouraging them to exercise through a daily walk, even when they don't feel like it. A survey of dog walkers reported that the exercise gave them a better overall sense of well-being and that even if they were feeling down, their mood improved once they were outside walking. Older dog walkers found that the exercise helped them stay physically fitter and maintain social contacts, and it encouraged children to spend more time outside and less time in front of the television or computer.

strange but true

A fitness trainer in California has devised a novel way for cat owners to integrate exercise into their day. Working out at home, having become bored with her sessions at the gym, Stephanie Jackson realised that at 3.6kg her cat, Bad, constituted the perfect piece of weight-training equipment. She devised a 30-minute workout involving exercises such as the Cat Crunch and the Dead-cat Lift. After a few months of daily cat-flexing, Jackson was amazed at the changes in both her own physique and that of her furry sidekick who had slimmed down considerably.

California now has regular cat-flexing competitions. Proponents have also tried flexing with other pets – anything from Yorkshire terriers to lizards. (And to those who suggest the practice is humiliating to animals, their retort is that it is an uplifting experience for your pet.)

did you know?

Dog owners who walk their dogs regularly are more active and have less body fat than non-dog owners, according to the American College of Sports Medicine. In a study looking at differences in physical activity levels and weight status, the ACSM found that dog owners fared better.

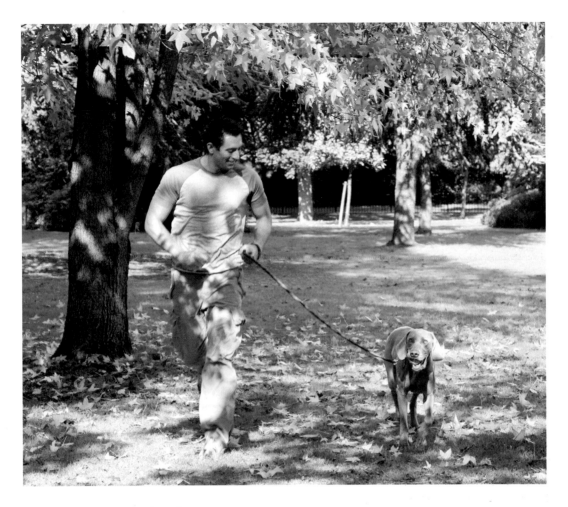

Integrated exercise for your podgy pooch

Dogs are not immune to the effects of their owners' sedentary lifestyles. In fact, according to America's National Academy of Sciences (NAS), around 25 per cent of canine pets in the West are overweight. Like humans, overweight dogs are more susceptible to injury and as their fat levels increase, so will their risk of developing cardiac problems, diabetes and arthritis. They will also experience more stress on their lungs, liver, kidneys and joints.

You can tell if your dog is overweight by checking to see if you can feel their ribs. If you cannot or if their waist isn't easily defined and if the dog appears to have a layer of fat on its tail, then it is too heavy. But what can you do about it?

Start by gently increasing the amount of activity your dog does while gradually decreasing its calorie intake. For unfit, overweight dogs, a daily 10-minute walk is a good starting point. Try playing more games with them too – throwing a frisbee or ball is an ideal way to monitor their activity levels and gradually increase them. The fitter they get, the more exercise they can handle. Don't think you are being kind to them by allowing them to become lazy.

gardening

Want to find an outdoor mind–body workout, but one that's within easy access of your home? Look no further than your own back garden. Pruning, weeding and tending to your lawns and flower beds can help to rid the body of tension in the same way as would a course of yoga.

In a three-year study, researchers found that gardening had a positive effect on the physical and emotional health of people with stress, depression or other mental health problems. People who spent time gardening had more time for reflection and relaxation, thereby improving their mood. Being outside in the fresh air, undertaking physical exercise and nurturing plants all helped to boost well-being and self-esteem. Environmental psychologists carrying out a similar study found that gardening reduces stress more effectively than many other methods of relaxation.

But gardening gives your body an excellent workout, too. Hauling and spreading compost and soil, moving plants and shrubs and raking and digging will make you break into a sweat and strengthen your muscles and bones at the same time. Reaching or bending to weed or plant is great for increasing your flexibility. And who needs a treadmill when you've got a lawnmower? (That's a push mower, of course!)

Back to nature

If you have back problems there are a few points you should bear in mind:

- Take gardening steadily as the strenuous exercise might exacerbate pain.
- Avoid getting too hot or cold while gardening as this can increase body stress.
- Use well-designed tools to lessen the risk of back pain (specially designed tools for people with back problems should be available at good garden centres).
- If you have a lot of trees in the garden, getting up the leaves can be a problem. There are excellent light-weight garden vacuums available that shred the leaves as they suck them in.

In fact, gardening uses almost every muscle in the body:

- Raking and leaf-sweeping use the pectoral muscles in the chest, the shoulder and back muscles

- Digging uses the quadriceps, hamstring and calf muscles in the legs as well as the triceps in the arms and back and trunk muscles

- Mowing uses the larger muscles in the legs and upper body, especially the arms

- Weeding and planting use the back and shoulder muscles

- Put it all together and you can burn as many calories in an hour's gardening as you would in a gym circuit (about 450)

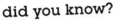

did you know?

The Green Gym in the UK, run by environmental group British Trust for Conservation Volunteers runs projects in green spaces for people to get involved in — and get fit at the same time. Many other European countries also run similar schemes. And it's not just volunteers who join; doctors refer people to the 'gyms' to help improve their health, lose weight or to recuperate.

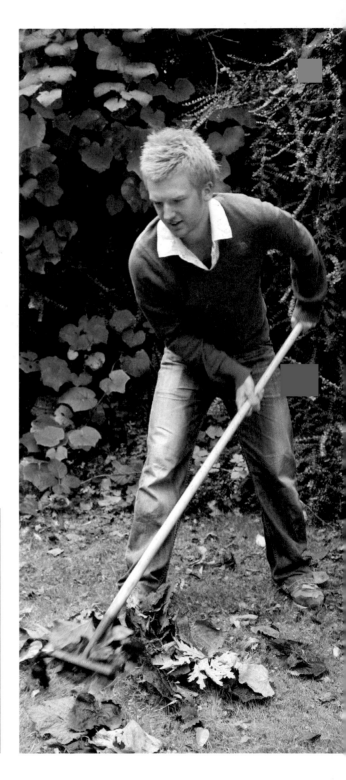

your gardening workout

Before you start, walk around your garden (or allotment) a few times, taking in some deep breaths.

Quad stretch

Standing with your feet hip-width apart, place your left hand on a tree or wall for support. Bend your right leg behind you, taking your ankle in your right hand and gently easing your foot towards your buttocks.

Hold for 5–10 seconds to stretch the hip and thigh muscles. Repeat with the other leg.

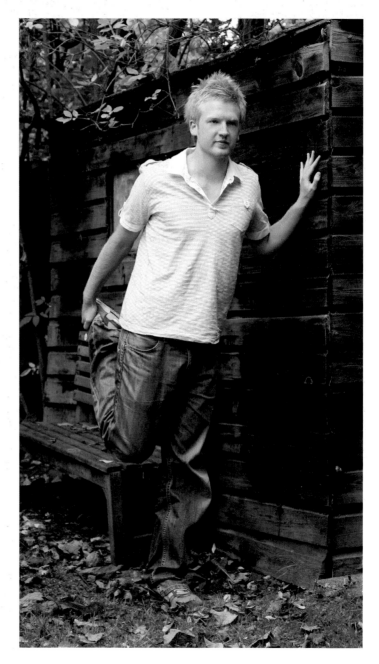

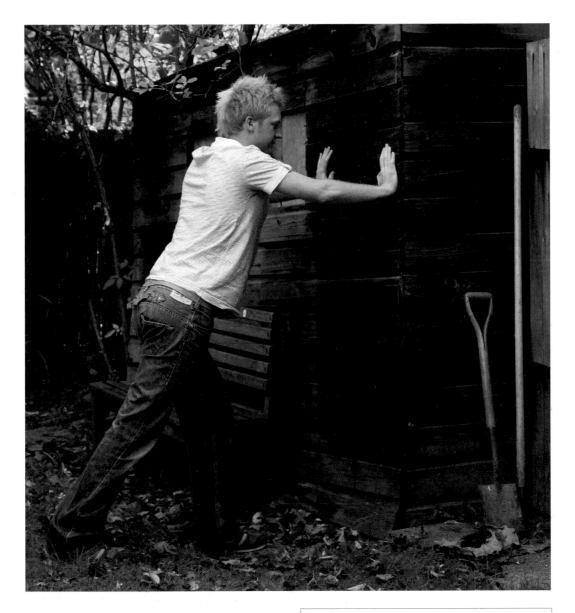

Calf stretch

Stand straight and tall, an arm's length away from a tree or wall. Now step backwards with one leg, pressing your heel to the floor. When your back foot is far enough away from the wall you will feel a stretch in your calf muscle.

Hold for 5–10 seconds and repeat with the other leg.

did you know?

The most energetic gardening activities in terms of calories used are digging and shovelling. If you spend 30 minutes on either of these, you could burn between 200 and 360 calories.

Shoulder stretch

Stand straight and tall. Now bend your knees slightly and tilt your pelvis under. Interlock your fingers and stretch your hands away from you. Keep your shoulders relaxed and feel your shoulder blades moving apart. This is a great stretch for the back and shoulders.

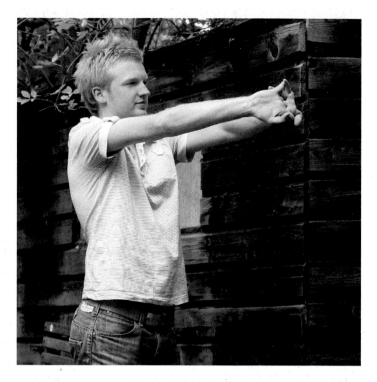

And remember...

If you are crouching down a lot, it is important to protect your back by standing up intermittently and gently arching backwards.

When pruning a bush, bend forwards from the waist and keep your back straight and bottom pushing out – it is far safer than having a rounded back and shoulders.

Break up particular tasks to avoid overusing one muscle group. Repeating the same movement over and over again will put your joints under strain.

If you crave nothing more than **slumping in front of the television after a day's gardening**, take note: the armchair is often the exhausted gardener's undoing. Injuries often occur when people slouch on the sofa in an awkward position, their posture out of line. Be conscious of how you are sitting if you don't want to end up like an ironing board the next day!

DIY fitness

Much like gardening and household cleaning chores, painting, decorating and putting together flat-pack furniture can constitute a tough workout. Here's how to get the most out of your DIY weekends:

Use conventional tools, rather than the high-tech, labour-saving variety wherever possible. A hand saw is cheaper than an electric one, for instance, it doesn't need replacement blades every few minutes and the exercise of sawing is great for the arms, chest and shoulders. Plumbing, painting and decorating involve a lot of squatting and climbing of ladders which is great for developing leg muscles. Try to keep equipment (such as tools and pots of paint) out of reach so that you have to walk to get them. Strenuous tasks such as sanding floorboards, laying concrete slabs, erecting fences or carrying bricks, cement or gravel are all great for simulating weight training. In fact, they are the equivalent of running in terms of their calorie-burning effects.

Stripping wallpaper can be tough work, especially if you are operating paper-stripping machinery and climbing up and down ladders. Half an hour of this activity will burn the same number of calories you would consume in three whiskies!

work it out

You may find it impossible to resist a **freshly cooked doughnut**, but do you know what you are guzzling as you lick the sugar from your lips? An average ring doughnut contains 140 calories and 2g of fat; make that a jam doughnut and you are looking at 250 calories and 19 per cent sugar. American imports with creamy fillings are especially unkind to your waistline with up to 390 calories and 12g of fat (4 of which are saturated). To work off even a plain ring doughnut you'd need to do one of the following:

- walk to a shop 28 minutes away at a moderate pace
- sweep up leaves and trim shrubs for 38 minutes
- clean out the garage for 38 minutes
- push a shopping trolley full of goods and containing a small child for 25 minutes
- wash and dry dishes for 45 minutes
- pick your own fruit and vegetables for 43 minutes.

chapter four

Many people – myself included – need no excuse to go shopping. But how about losing pounds as you spend them? Because shopping is done on foot (unless you are an on-line shopping addict), it provides the ideal opportunity for integrating some extra gusto as you gaze longingly in the windows of your favourite exclusive boutique or even as you push the trolley during your weekly supermarket shop.

integrated exercise at the shops

Parking as far as possible from the shop and carrying your bags to the car instead of using a trolley is just one important part of your shopping workout; the exercises below will complete it.

Trolley lunges

A study at San Diego State University showed that the walking lunge is one of the most effective ways to firm your bottom.

1 Begin by standing with feet together, keeping your hands on the trolley. Keep your back upright, tummy muscles tucked in and face directly ahead.

2 Take a long step forwards, being careful not to extend your knee over your toes. Your left leg should be extended behind you with the knee slightly flexed.

3 Squeeze the buttocks as you push off your front (right) leg to step forwards again.

Repeat this lunge walking for the full length of one aisle.

Trolley squats

This works the gluteal muscles that shape your bottom and the quadriceps at the front of the thighs.

1 Holding on to your trolley, stand with your feet shoulder-width apart and your tummy muscles tucked in.

2 Slowly lower yourself into a squat until your thighs are parallel to the ground. Don't let your knees extend beyond your toes and push your bottom out as you get lower. Slowly return to the upright position.

Repeat 10 times.

Shopping trolley row

This will help develop your triceps muscles (at the back of your upper arm).

1 Push your shopping trolley with both arms fully extended. The weight of the trolley will put a static contraction on.

2 Every so often pull the trolley in and push out in a sort of rowing action to work all the muscles in the upper body.

Baked bean biceps curls

This will firm the front of your upper arms and forearms.

1 Stand with your hands shoulder-width apart and with a tin of baked beans in each one, palms facing upwards. Keeping your back straight, your chest lifted and your tummy muscles tucked in, till your `pelvis forwards.

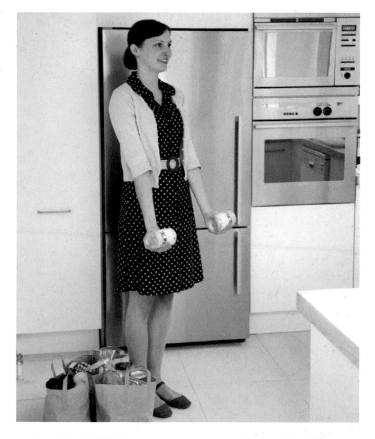

2 Tuck your elbows into your body and keep your wrists straight as you slowly raise the tins up to shoulder height. It is important to keep elbows tucked in as you do this. Hold briefly and then lower the tins back down to the start position.

Repeat 10 times.

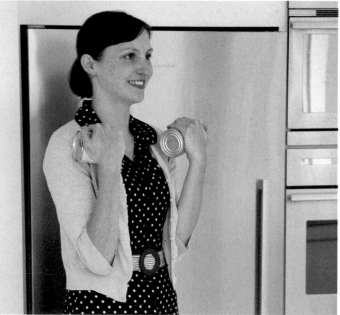

Shopping-bag raise

Here is an exercise to help tone the muscles in your arms, chest and shoulders.

1 Stand with two evenly weighted shopping bags by your sides. Bend your knees to pick up the bags by their handles and slowly stand up, but don't straighten your legs completely.

2 Making sure you are stable with your back straight and head facing forwards, slowly lift the bags so your arms are raised out from your sides, almost parallel to the floor. Don't lock your elbows fully. Hold for a second or two before lowering the bags back down.

Repeat 5 times.

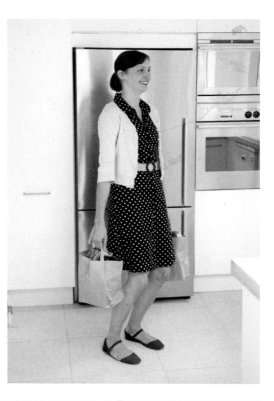

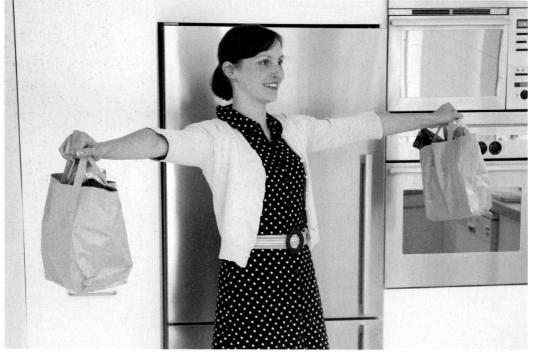

Baguette side stretch

This tones the waist area. You will need a large French stick or baguette to do it!

1 Stand with your feet shoulder-width apart and hold the baguette above your head with one hand at each end. Your knees should be slightly bent to ensure a stable base.

2 Keeping your back straight, shoulders and hips facing forwards and your head and neck in line with the torso, lean carefully and slowly to the right. You should feel a gentle stretch in the sides of your trunk and waist. Hold for a few seconds, then return to the upright position.

Repeat 6 times on each side.

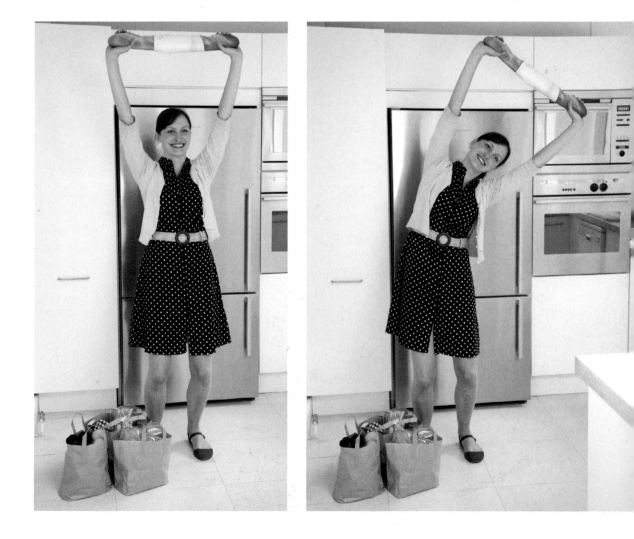

Losing pounds from your thighs, not your pocket, is precisely the idea behind mall-walking (also known as 'mallercise'), a fitness craze that is already hugely popular in America and is rapidly catching on in Europe. Mall-walking workouts are now so popular in the States and in Canada that the shoe manufacturer Hush Puppies even markets a special shoe 'to give extra traction for smoother, slicker mall floors'.

As its name suggest, the activity involves power-walking around indoor shopping malls, making use of stairs and escalators (stepping up them, of course) as well as the wide concourses that feature in many of the centres. The advantages (besides the fact that you get to window shop as you walk) are that shopping malls are traffic free (and therefore fume free), weather resistant (so you can wear what you like without worrying about the likelihood of a sudden downpour) and usually quite safe.

Researchers looking at the specific benefits of mall-walking have found it to be beneficial to both body and mind. At the University of Calgary, physiologists looked at the effects of an eight-week mall-walking programme on health and well-being. At the end of it subjects were found to be walking further and to weigh less than when they started. Perhaps more encouragingly, they displayed high self-motivation with 63 per cent of them mall-walking on three or more days a week. Also,

the average age of the subjects was sixty-six which led the researchers to suggest that this is the perfect activity for all ages, particularly for older people looking for a safe, flat place to improve their functional mobility, fitness and sense of independence.

Make the most of your mall-walking

Walk with a friend (whose fitness level is similar to yours) or join a mall-walking group (ask for details at major shopping centres – see page 160). You could also mall-walk with your baby in a buggy.

Choose a time when the mall is relatively free of customers. Mornings may be better than late-night shopping evenings, for instance.

Make sure you **wear comfortable shoes**. Trainers or cross-trainers are ideal.

Load **motivational music** onto your iPod or MP3 player so you can listen to good 'walking' songs as you stride.

Set personal goals: decide when and how to increase the frequency, duration or intensity of your walks, then go for it. It may help to keep a journal to chart your progress so you can see how much you've accomplished.

Reward yourself: stop for a low-fat Americano coffee, fruit smoothie or low-fat yoghurt; get a massage; or splash out on that new outfit!

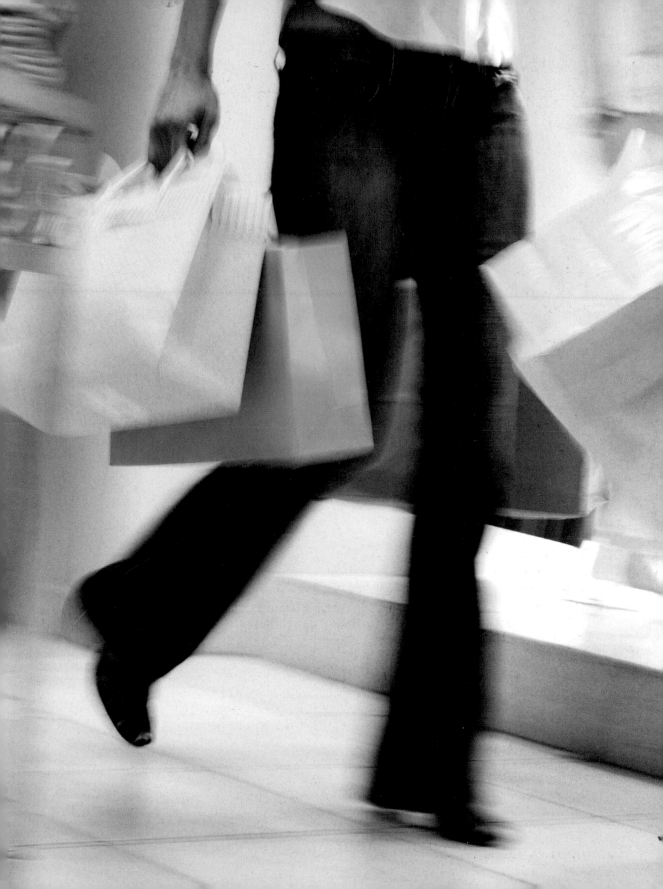

Warm up

Walk for 5 minutes at a pace that allows you to chat but at which you get warm. Use your arms to propel you along (see page 91 for details on correct walking technique).

'Mallercise'

Walk briskly for 5 minutes to the point where you are breathing quite heavily. Climb up staircases and escalators and weave in and out of other shoppers if you have to.

Cool down

Walk for 5 minutes at a slower pace to cool down.

Progression

As you get fitter, increase the length and intensity of the mallercise phase. Your ultimate aim should be to do a 5-minute warm up, 20-minutes mallercise and a 5-minute cool down.

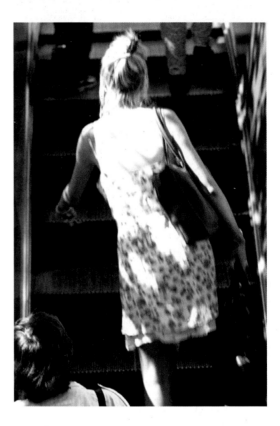

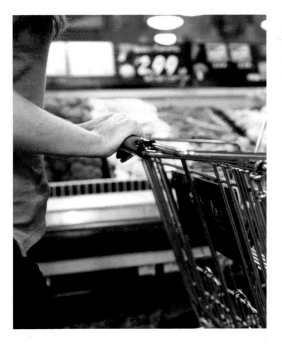

Pizzas are not necessarily unhealthy if you select a thin crust piled up with peppers, tomatoes, mushrooms and lean ham. High-fat toppings such as cheese and pepperoni add more calories and fat: a 9-inch four seasons pizza has 900 calories; a pepperoni, cheese and tomato has 1040; and a deep-pan, meat-topped pizza with cheese-filled crust contains almost 2000 calories. Frozen pizzas bought at supermarkets tend have more weight in the base and less in toppings resulting in fewer calories. So, to burn off an average 790 calories in a plain cheese and tomato pizza you would have to do one of the following:

- walk a total of 3 hours during the day
- carry a backpack while shopping for 97 minutes
- climb up and down stairs for 90 minutes
- take the kids ice skating or roller-blading for 2 hours and 20 minutes
- dance while doing the housework for 2 hours and 30 minutes
- assemble flat-pack furniture for 2 hours and 30 minutes.

strange but true

A high-tech trolley has been manufactured to transform supermarket shopping into a gentle workout. Shoppers are thought to burn up about 160 calories during a typical 40-minute visit to the supermarket, but pushing the Trim Trolley for the same time with the resistance level set at seven (ten being the hardest) the average person would use up 280 calories. That's the equivalent of calories burned during a 20-minute swim at a leisurely pace and about double the amount used when walking for 40 minutes.

The shopper sets the Trim Trolley to different levels of 'shopping resistance', making it harder or easier to push, and the trolley monitors heart rate, number of calories burned and when the shopper starts to burn fat instead of carbohydrates.

chapter five

Of all the exercise forms that can be integrated into your daily life, the ones in this chapter are among the best for boosting cardiovascular health and calorie burning as well as the most practical. Incorporate them whenever and wherever you can, getting the most from them by using them as part of a 'commutathon' – a means of getting yourself efficiently and effectively from A to B, be that work, the shops or the school run and back.

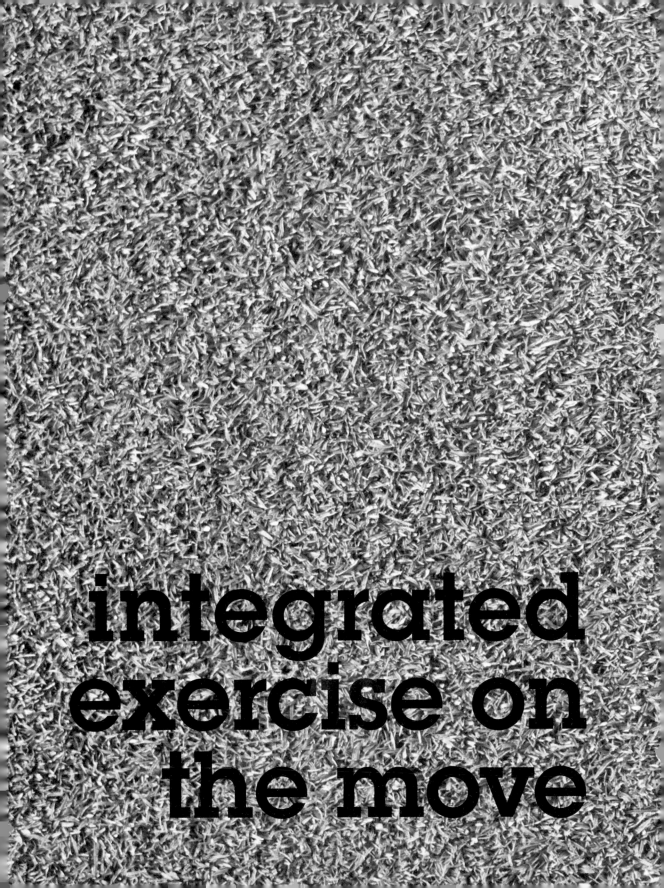

integrated
exercise on
the move

every second counts

It is staggering to think that around 70 per cent of people in Europe live within 6 miles of their workplace, yet most travel to and from work by car, train or bus. Imagine a journey that did not involve the stress of traffic jams, congestion, roadworks and hold-ups, and which enabled you to arrive at work feeling fitter, healthier and calmer.

If walking, in-line skating or jogging to your workplace are completely impractical, why not consider using the 'park and ride' or 'park and walk' facilities in your area? Simply park a little farther away from the office and cycle or walk the last 10 or 15 minutes. Remember that every second and minute count towards your daily total of integrated exercise points.

did you know?
Commuting by car and train has been scientifically linked to higher blood pressure, greater degrees of tension, reduced performance in specific jobs and bad moods at the end of the working day. Other physical side effects include stiff necks, excessive tiredness and lower-back pain.

did you know?
'Walking is as close to a magic bullet as you'll find in modern medicine. If there was a pill that could lower the risk of chronic disease like walking does, then people would be clamouring for it.'
JoAnn Manson, Professor of Medicine at Harvard University

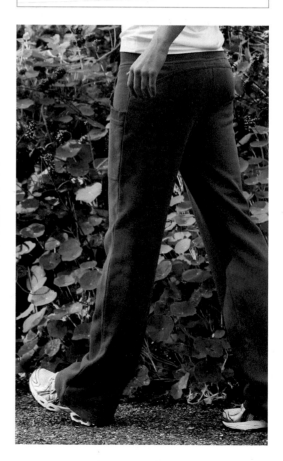

walking

This is an activity requiring no gym subscription and no spandex, Lycra or legwarmers, and it is one to which even the most fitness-phobic individual might not be averse. A daily stroll is predicted to become the favourite means of getting fit over the next decade, suggesting we will be taking to the pavements in hordes, akin to the jogging boom of the 1970s. Integrate walking into your day and not only will the pounds melt away, you will feel and look better.

I find it helps to view walking as a mode of transport – a means to an end. Instead of taking the car, I power-walk my son to his nursery, walk to the local shops instead of using the supermarket a few miles away and walk my dog every day. These are all things I need to get done – but I am getting fit while doing them.

Body benefits

Walking uses much the same muscles as running – it strengthens the hamstring, quadriceps, iliopsoas muscles at the front of the hips, calf and the gluteus maximus muscles with each stride – but is far kinder to the joints. Physical benefits of regular walking range from lowering the risk of gallstones and stroke to reducing sleep problems. A broader set of disorders – from sexual dysfunction to cognitive decline – can also be alleviated by a brisk walk around the block. For instance, researchers found walking prevented peripheral artery disease which impairs blood flow in the legs and causes leg pain in one-fifth of elderly people.

Of course, walking also helps you to lose weight. Scientists revealed that overweight people who walked briskly for 30–60 minutes a day lost 3kg in about eighteen months even if they didn't change any other lifestyle habits. Another study found that people who walked at least 4 hours a week gained an average of 4kg less in weight than their sedentary counterparts with age. A leisurely walk (at 2mph) was also found to be the best formula to help obese people shed pounds.

Mind benefits

The ability to maintain some level of daily walking has been termed the most accurate predictor of illness and death in elderly people. Comparing the effects of a walking programme over a toning and stretching regime in elderly subjects, researchers found that walkers performed far better in tests of mental agility. Like other forms of aerobic exercise, it increases oxygen supplies and blood flow to the brain, helping it to stay more alert and work more efficiently.

Walking can also improve memory and prevent memory loss. A study of more than 2,200 Japanese–American men aged between 71 and 93 showed that those who were sedentary or who walked less than 0.4km a day were nearly twice as likely to develop dementia and Alzheimer's disease compared with those who walked more than 3.2km every day.

Perfect your technique

You won't walk your way to fitness if you are dawdling along, staring at the pavement. Instead, stand tall, arms by your sides and pull your navel towards your spine so that your core muscles are working. Focus your eyes 5–6 metres ahead and keep your shoulders relaxed. Bend your elbows to a 90-degree angle and cup your hands lightly, rather than clenching your fists. Leading with the heel, take a step forwards with your right foot and move your arms in opposition (i.e. as your left arm moves forwards, the right moves back). Transfer your weight through the heel of your right foot. A common mistake is to allow the arms to swing from side to side rather than backwards and forwards. Walking with straight, rigid arms is another bad practice. It is much harder to walk at any speed without the propelling motion of the arms.

How far to walk

Accumulating 10,000 steps daily (about 8km) is recommended as a healthy threshold by many leading fitness experts (most people in the West walk only 4,500 steps a day). In order to lose a significant amount of weight you would probably need to tot up at least 16,000 steps a day if walking was your sole form of exercise.

Measuring your steps accurately can be tricky. Pedometers are useful tools, but a study in the *British Journal of Sports Medicine* found the very cheapest pedometers overestimated the number of steps taken by as much as 1034 per cent. Of around a thousand pedometers tested, only a quarter gave measurements within an 'acceptable' 10 per cent margin of error. If you plan to make walking the mainstay of your integrated exercise plan, then a pedometer is a useful piece of equipment to invest in, but go for a mid-range product, not the bargain-basement variety.

Where to walk

There is little doubt that walking anywhere at all is beneficial, but if you have the chance to vary the terrain, so much the better. Adding hills to your route, for instance, will speed up your burning off calories. Your heart rate will rise going uphill, while downhill you really have to contract your leg muscles to work against gravity and slow your descent. Walking on softer surfaces, such as mud, sand or grass, also means you use more energy than you would walking on concrete or tarmac because your leg muscles need to work harder to push upwards and forwards for each step.

Walking on cobblestones, or as rocky ground as you can find, may have even more profound benefits. Physiologists found cobblestone-walking, an activity rooted in traditional Chinese medicine, leads to significant reductions in blood pressure and improvements in balance. It is thought that the uneven surfaces may stimulate acupressure points on the soles of the feet, thereby regulating blood pressure. Because it is challenging, it will also burn more calories.

Nordic walking

For even faster weight-loss results, you could try Nordic walking (or 'urban trekking' as it is known in the USA). The idea is to hike through the urban jungle with two ski-like poles which, despite looking suspect, does have proven benefits. Professor John Pocari, an exercise physiologist at the University of Wisconsin, found that the use of walking poles forces people to pick up their pace and work harder without realising it. The fact alone that you are using your arms through a greater range of motion than normal means you are increasing calorie expenditure.

six great ways to integrate walking into your day

1 Carry your baby in a sling and head out for a stroll.

2 Identify a coffee shop 10 minutes away and power-walk there and back during your lunch hour.

3 Walk on the spot every time you talk on the phone.

4 Get up early and walk either to the train station or bus stop or the entire route to work.

5 Go mall walking at weekends or during your lunch hour (see page 84).

6 Get a dog – the best way to ensure that you get your daily stroll (see page 70).

did you know?
Researchers from the University of Exeter reported that just 5–10 minutes of walking a day can significantly cut cravings for cigarettes among people trying to kick the habit.

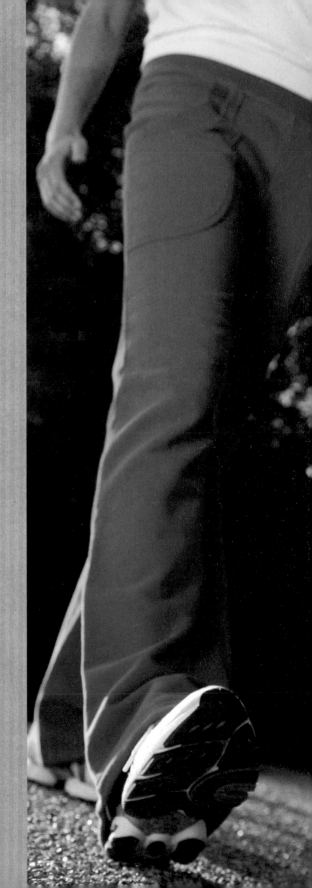

go retro

If you find jogging or walking a bit boring, how about doing it backwards? Running (or walking) backwards – retro-running as it is known among enthusiasts – has few obvious attractions to the casual observer, yet an increasing number of people who try it claim it gives their activity regime a whole new perspective.

Body benefits

Remarkably, scientists have discovered there are some distinct benefits to this bizarre activity. Retro-running dates back to the 1970s when a small group of physiotherapists began recommending it to injured athletes and footballers. Because it involves less movement of the hips the impact on the joints decreases, making it an ideal form of rehabilitation for someone with knee and back problems. A South African study found backward training also improved cardio-respiratory fitness while helping to streamline the physique of a group of novice runners.

Getting started

This requires some planning. You should start somewhere safe such as a track or familiar road where you will avoid potholes, road signs and other hazards. Go slowly, taking small steps at first, staying in control. Let the ball of the foot contact first, then allow the heel to touch just briefly. If this feels all right, repeat the 1-minute backwards segments two or three times, jogging forwards slowly in-between.

Perfect your technique

After a few weeks you will feel less anxious about collisions and can begin to step up your retro-running to 5 or 6 minutes in total. At this point, you can try taking longer steps and, if you want to stretch your legs more, try running backwards on a slightly downward slope.

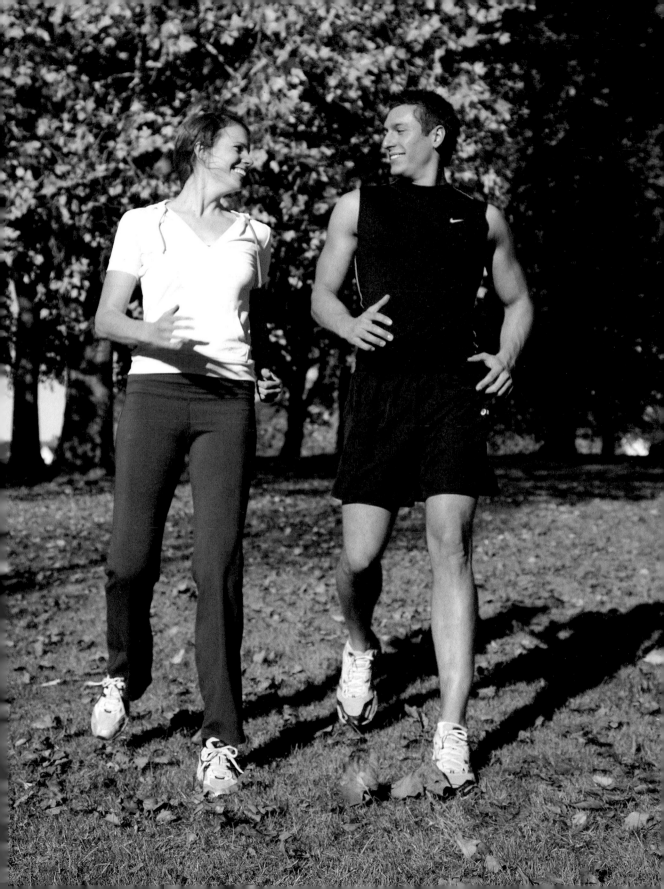

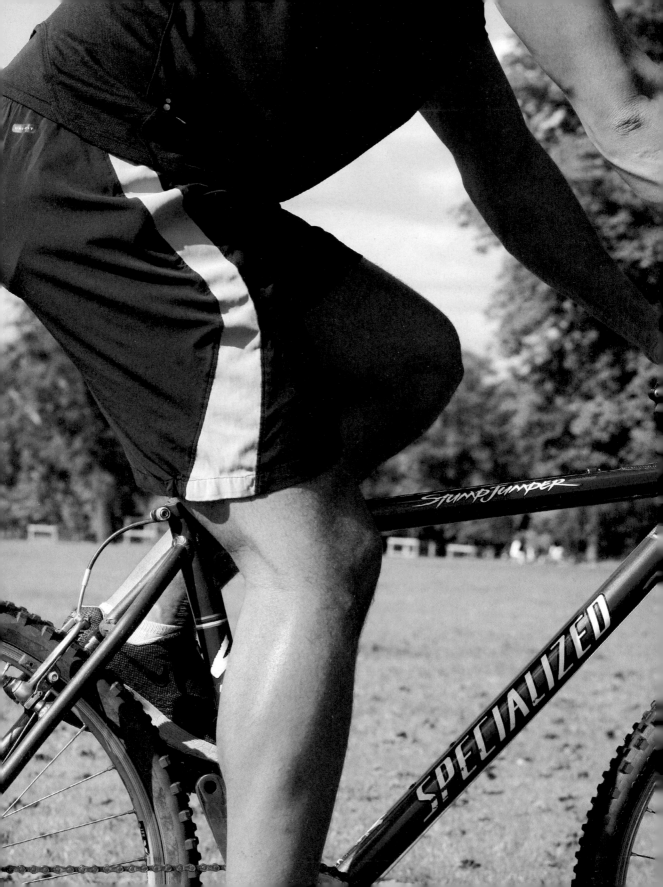

cycling

Getting on your bike to go to work is one of the most effective routes to stress relief as well as weight loss. As cars and buses reach a standstill in traffic jams, you can just sail past in the cycling lane, smug in the knowledge that you will not only get to your destination more quickly, but will be toning your legs and bottom, as well as improving your heart health in the process. And the advantages don't end there. For most commuters who normally take the car, a commute by bike would save the equivalent of the weight of a small car in CO_2 emissions every year.

Body benefits

Pedalling works most of the muscles in the legs and buttocks during the pushdown phase so it will give you an unbelievably toned lower body. But your heart and lungs are the biggest beneficiaries if you cycle regularly. You will also burn calories – even coasting at 3mph burns 2 calories a minute. Increase the pace and cover undulating terrain and you are looking at burning at least 400 calories an hour.

However, since your body is supported by the bike, cycling is classed a non-weight-bearing activity and therefore won't strengthen bones to protect against osteoporosis as much as walking or running do. Some researchers suggest cycling won't do much for male virility either with studies showing a link between cycling and reduced blood flow, leading to erectile dysfunction. Narrow, unpadded seats were found to cause the most problems and a wide variety of more comfortable alternatives is now available for men. But the benefits of cycling far outweigh the pitfalls, so get out there and do it!

Getting started

Obviously you will need a bike. Go to a specialist shop for advice about appropriate saddles and the best size of bike for you. Padded cycling shorts are essential for comfort and to prevent chafing if you plan to cycle a significant distance to work. If you haven't cycled in a while, regain your confidence by starting with a 10- or 20-minute ride on flat terrain and build up gradually over a month until you can keep going for longer.

Perfect your technique

Make sure your seat is positioned correctly – a common mistake made by novice cyclists is to set it too high or too low which reduces pedal power. Your extended leg at the bottom of the pedal stroke should be almost straight to avoid cramps and improve efficiency. Don't use too high or low a gear, as you will only expend unnecessary effort – aim for around 60–70 revolutions per minute to maximise blood flow to the lower limbs.

running

Running is the most natural of movements. From toddlerhood onwards, the quickest way for a human being to get anywhere under their own steam is to run. But it has other advantages that go far beyond just being a means of transport. For one thing it is one of the most effective ways of burning fat and getting fit.

Body benefits

The basic running action strengthens the hamstring, quadriceps, iliopsoas muscles at the front of the hips and the calf and gluteus maximus muscles with each stride, while the pumping action of your arms strengthens the upper body to some extent. Around 590 calories will be gobbled up if you run at 6mph (a 10-minute mile), even more as you get faster. Generally, you will burn more calories running off road as your legs have to work harder on soft ground.

Running is a higher-impact activity than walking which means it is not so good for protecting vulnerable joints and, as such, may not be suitable for everyone. Each time a jogger's foot strikes the ground, a shock equivalent to three times their body weight reverberates from their feet, through their legs and into their spine.

Getting started

One of the biggest advantages of running to work is that there is little financial outlay required. It is important to choose well-cushioned running shoes from a specialist shop and, for women, a good sports bra, but otherwise you can wear pretty much anything that is comfortable enough to allow a full range of movement for your arms and legs when you run. Swanky gear may look good, but an old pair of jogging bottoms will do the job just as well.

Perfect your technique

You don't have to be a rocket scientist to figure out that because the average head weighs about 4.5kg, its nodding movement is going to place a tremendous load on the rest of the body while running, creating tension in the shoulders and putting pressure on the spine. Focusing your gaze around 20–30 metres ahead can help to keep your head in a steady position. Foot-slapping (or running flat-footed – more common on treadmills as people struggle to adjust their foot patterns) is a warning sign that something is wrong with your technique – you are literally jarring your whole system – so practise running lightly and quietly, landing on the balls of your feet rather than on your heels. Another common mistake is allowing your hands to flop. Far from being more relaxing, this actually creates tension, as the shoulders tighten to pick up the slack.

five great ways to integrate running into your day

1 Run when you could walk – break into a gentle jog when you are walking the dog, walking to work or even pushing your child in their buggy.

2 Find out if there are running groups at or near your workplace. If not, set one up. Integrating a run into your day can do wonders for your work output.

3 If you already walk to work, set yourself mini challenges such as running between alternate lamp posts. Variations in speed between running and walking (a practice known in Swedish as 'fartlek' meaning 'speed play') can have profound effects on fitness levels.

4 Run up and down stairs instead of walking.

5 Run in water. It may sound bizarre, but if you have time to get to a pool, then invest in a buoyancy belt to keep you afloat as you go for a deep-water jog. Physiotherapists recommend it as an impact-free way to stay fit and strong.

did you know?

Conventional wisdom puts running as an enemy of the hips and knees. However, the results of a study showed that, rather than inflicting wear and tear, regular running protects vulnerable joints from damage and pain. An American research team followed more than 500 runners from a local club (called 'ever runners' in the study) and 300 inactive people ('never runners', but not necessarily sedentary) in their fifties and sixties for 14 years.

When results from an annual health questionnaire were analysed, it was found that:

- 'ever runners', who ran at least 6 hours a week on average, experienced less pain and injuries by the time they were in their sixties and seventies than the 'never runners'.

- whereas 43 per cent of the inactive group had arthritis, only 35 per cent of the joggers were found to suffer from the condition.

It seems that the protective effect stemmed from consistency of running which helped to build strong bones, joints and tendons.

stair-climbing

Ever wondered where the inspiration for one of the gym's best-used and most effective items of fitness equipment came from? The answer is something you almost certainly use every day – the stairs. Stairclimber machines are based on the principles of walking (or running) up ordinary flights of stairs, an activity so physically testing that it is included in the training regimes of professional athletes, boxers and footballers.

Body benefits

It is not only the butt-firming, leg-toning, stomach-flattening effects of regular stair-climbing that make it one of the best forms of exercise around. Sports scientists from Northern Ireland found that walking up stairs for an average of 6 minutes a day can lower cholesterol by 10–15 per cent and make you 10–15 per cent fitter. Their research looked at the effects of intermittently climbing a few flights of stairs and discovered that cardiovascular fitness and health were significantly enhanced.

Another study involved workers using the stairs rather than a lift for 6 weeks, at the end of which the overweight employees in particular were found to have lost significant amounts of weight.

Technique

Keep your back straight and hips facing forwards. Bend your arms at right angles and pump them to get up the stairs. Do not twist your head or back as you step.

How many stairs should you aim to climb?

Climbing three flights of stairs a day is better than none. According to Sport England's Everyday Sport campaign which recommends stair-climbing as an excellent route to fitness, climbing 3,407m of stairs is the equivalent of climbing three small mountains! Now that's something to aim for!

did you know?

A Harvard University study found that men who climbed, on average, at least eight flights of stairs a day had a 33 per cent lower mortality rate than men who were sedentary.

strange but true

Skyscraper stair-climbs are the latest fitness challenge in Chicago, Boston, Denver, Detroit, Toronto, Miami and San Francisco, while in the Big Apple the New York Road Runners group has staged an annual since 1978. Backed by the American Lung Association, these stair-climbing fundraisers appeal because they offer a cardio-lung workout that can provide the same benefits in 15 minutes as those you would get from running for twice as long on level ground.

car exercises

If you do have to travel by car, make sure you stay as active as you safely can by doing some of these exercises while you drive.

Buttock clenching

This tones the gluteal muscles and can be done pretty much anywhere unnoticed. Simply squeeze together the buttock muscles for 10 seconds and then release. Repeat 10 times.

Thigh toning

As you drive, squeeze together your inner thighs. You can make this more effective by placing something between your legs (a tennis ball or jumper, for instance). Hold each squeeze for 10 seconds and repeat 10 times.

Shoulder release

As you hold the steering wheel, lower your shoulders and pull back as if you are trying to position a coin between your shoulder blades. Hold for 10 seconds and release. Do not pull on the steering wheel when you do this – it should be held lightly.

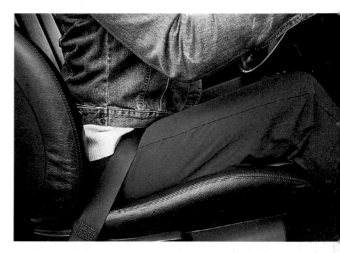

work it out

Feeling thirsty and think grabbing a cola is the answer? Not so fast. Very **fizzy drinks** are high in sugar unless they contain artificial sweeteners and a regular 330ml can of cola provides an unhealthy 35.6g of sugar and 141.8 calories per serving. To burn off that one can you'd need to do one of the following:

- be a cheerleader at a sports match for 23.5 minutes
- act in a play for 28 minutes
- clean gutters for 30 minutes
- run up stairs carrying a full suitcase for 14 minutes.

in-line skating

In-line skating has a reputation for being among the coolest and most fashionable modes of transport. But don't let its trendy image put you off trying it. This is an activity that is suitable for anyone of any age, from teenagers to octogenarians. It's worthwhile getting some practice in, or even having some lessons, before you use it as a commuter activity and glide your way to a more streamlined body.

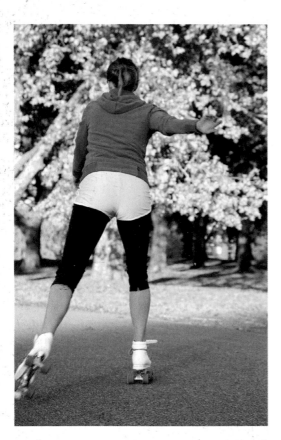

Body benefits

Although the aerobic benefits of gliding along on a pair of skates are not colossal, they are still greater than you would get from driving or taking a train to work. And with a bit of effort, skating can be transformed into a tough workout with bursts of speed, lunges and other exercises performed on wheels. Your leg and buttock muscles obviously benefit most (Kylie Minogue claimed her pert bottom is a result of regular in-line skating). It is low impact, so great for anyone with weak knees. And you can burn up to 380 calories an hour.

Getting started

You will need a pair of skates and protective gear for your head, elbows, hands and knees. Although helmets aren't compulsory, they are a useful safety precaution if you plan skating in areas where there is a high volume of traffic and you have to cross roads frequently on your journey. If you are a novice, it is highly recommended that you hire some skates before forking out to buy the equipment. Remember, there are limitations as to where you can skate – it is banned in some places – so check the rules in and around your local area before you take off.

Perfect your technique

Even if you can skate already, it is worth having lessons to perfect your technique (these are held in many parks). A bit like skiing, the technique of in-line skating requires you to position your knees slightly in front of your toes, with your shins pressing down on to the front of the boots. Imagine you are pushing a pram when you skate (swinging your arms will throw you off balance) and start with your feet hip-width apart. From there, try 'scooting' along by pushing one skate directly to the side, then pulling it all the way back in.

Make it harder

Skate-tuck-roll: this is a great way to strengthen thigh muscles. As you skate, bring your feet together. Bend your knees so that you sit into a deep squat. Place your hands on your knees and, keeping your back straight, hold this position for 5–10 seconds as you roll forwards. Skate normally for a few seconds then repeat.

did you know?

In-line skating has become so popular among city dwellers that the Pari-roller, a 30-km skating event held every Friday evening through the streets of Paris now attracts 15,000 competitors a week. Similar events are staged in London throughout the summer, as well as elsewhere in Europe and in the USA.

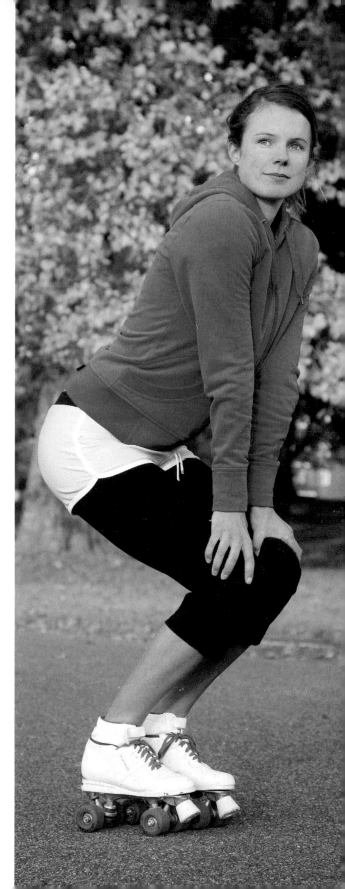

chapter six

Having children is often cited as one of the main reasons why people allow their fitness routines to wane. Family life can be frenetic and for parents who are trying to juggle everything – in many cases that means work, the school run, the children's social diaries as well as their own – there is precious little time to do anything other than collapse on the sofa at the end of the day. However, it may be far easier to integrate exercise into your day than you think. In fact, rather than blaming your children for your expanding waistline, you need only change your perspective, so that your children (and their lifestyles) become your gym.

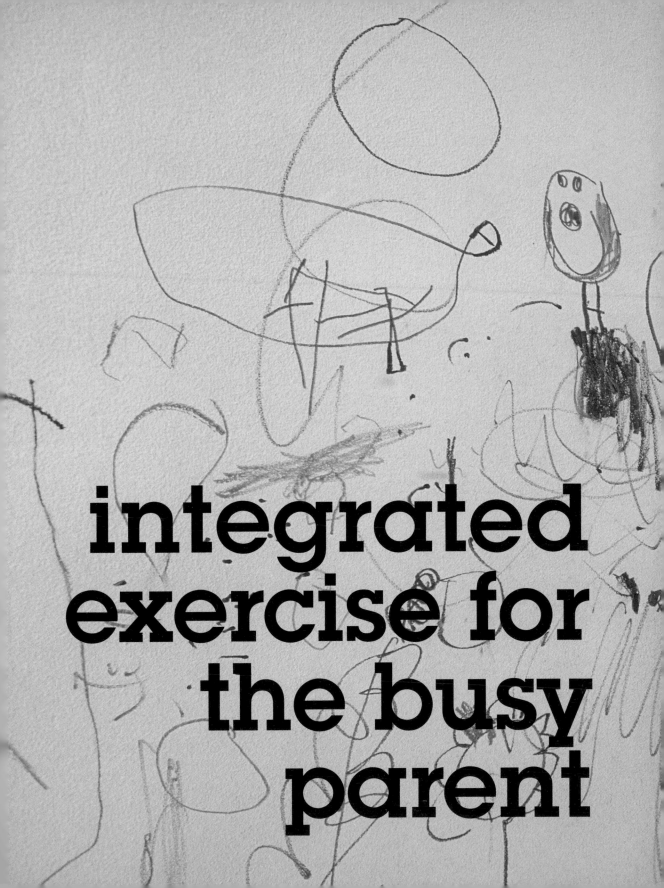

integrated
exercise for
the busy
parent

baby-flexing

Losing weight after you have a baby is hard enough without having to arrange for childcare so you can go to the gym or out for a run. So, the best news of all is that you can integrate exercise with your baby. Exercising together can make getting back in shape more fun and you get to spend quality time with your newborn. Here are some tips on how to get moving during those tentative first few weeks and months.

Equipment

New mums are constantly throwing buggies in and out of their cars, lifting bags full of baby paraphernalia, hauling high chairs about. Life itself suddenly becomes one long workout. Often, though, they do this without much attention to their body mechanics which can suffer adversely unless care is taken. The correct technique to lift a pushchair (which can be surprisingly heavy) is to make sure that you use your legs – don't bend at the waist which means you use your back muscles.

Baby carriers

Walking is one of the best forms of exercise and carrying your baby in a sling or carrier means added weight which will help you to burn more calories. Front carriers also leave your arms free so that you can do household chores and other jobs.

However, a lot of baby slings/carriers are not ergonomically sound and while they are good for the baby, they are not always so good for their parents. Most put the burden of

weight on the shoulders, which places stress on the joints and can throw the spine off balance. Unfortunately, front carriers also tend to pull the adult even further forwards encouraging a hunched-shoulder posture; this causes shortening of the chest muscles and weakening of the back muscles.

Happily, exercises with your baby in the carrier can offset these adverse effects. Try scapular contractions where you squeeze your shoulder blades together as if cracking a walnut to help pull your shoulders back and give your back the strength it needs. And remember, you should always carry baby in the front carrier with a strong, tall spine, shoulders pulled back and abdominal muscles pulled in.

did you know?

Just putting on some music can inspire you to do more activity. Research at London's Brunel University found that fast-beat music can lift a person's activity levels by as much as 20 per cent. Athletes who ran while listening to 'synchronous' music — in which the beats fitted with the rhythm of body movement — endured a fifth more exertion than those who didn't. Music heard 'asynchronously' (in the background) also acts to arouse a person and enhance their physical performance by as much as 10 per cent.

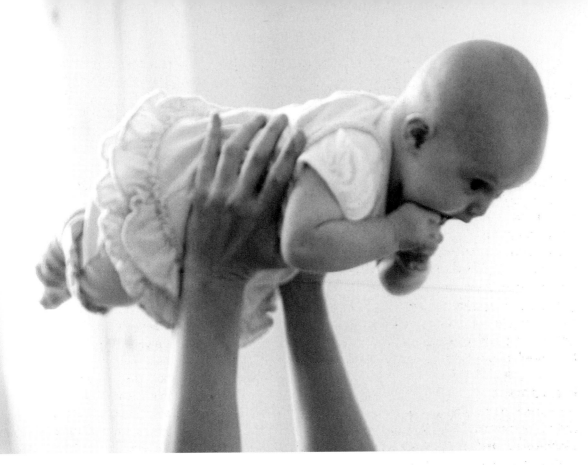

Holding baby

New babies love to be held. And mums will hold them in any way, shape or fashion that will allow them to still go about their daily life. Before long, though, this can result in back, hip and shoulder pain. Often, the underlying cause is holding the baby predominantly on one side of the body. Imagine the contortion that the spine must go through to repeatedly support both parent and baby in this position. Rather, try a position where baby is carried in the centre of your body so that your spine stays straight and strong and your baby's weight is distributed more evenly. This way, you use the muscles of your arm, rather than relying on your shoulders and joints. Failing that, simply switch sides regularly to avoid muscular imbalances that will ultimately affect posture.

strange but true

A tickling or joke-telling session with the children may help you get into shape. Laughing really does constitute a workout of sorts, say chartered physiotherapists, because it recruits the traversus abdominus, a muscle that helps to flatten the stomach area. Because it is so deeply embedded, however, it is difficult to target and a lot of fitness activities, like aerobics, don't work the abdominal area effectively. The real key to strengthening the traversus abdominus muscle lies in very subtle movements; laughing is ideal because it contracts the muscle appropriately.

Baby press-ups

This is a good way to strengthen the abdominal muscles weakened through childbirth; keep them tight while doing this exercise. Start with the half press-up (keeping your knees on the floor) and progress with the full press-up as you get stronger. Watch your baby giggle with pleasure as your face gets closer to them and then moves away again.

1 Lay your baby on the bed and get into the press-up position over the top of them, your hands beneath your shoulders and knees bent.

2 Slowly lower yourself down until your nose almost touches your baby's. Press your palms into the floor, straightening your arms and keeping your head, neck, back and hips in line as you lift your body back away from the bed.

Repeat 10–15 times, remembering to keep your abdominal muscles tight.

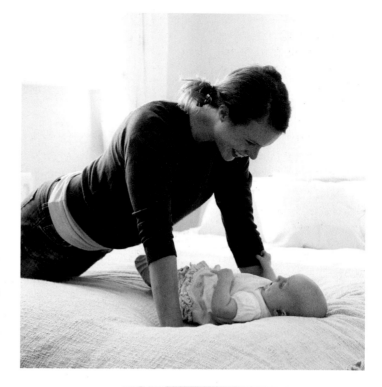

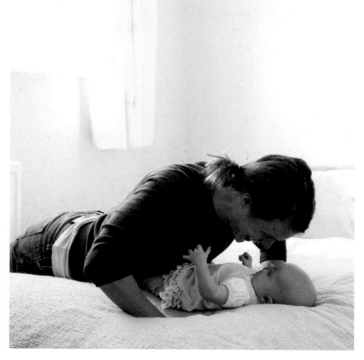

Baby-lifting

Who needs the gym when you have a baby who is the perfect little weight and will conveniently grow as your own muscles get stronger? These are great exercises for strengthening all the major muscles in the upper body; try them once your baby is strong enough to hold their own head (usually at around six months).

1 Lie on the bed holding your baby above you.

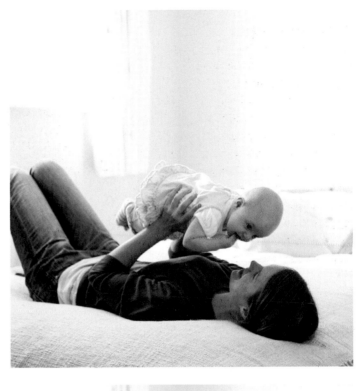

2 Gently lift your baby up in the air and bring them back down again. The slower and more controlled your lifting the more your muscles have to work.

Stand up and do the same thing, lifting your baby over your head.

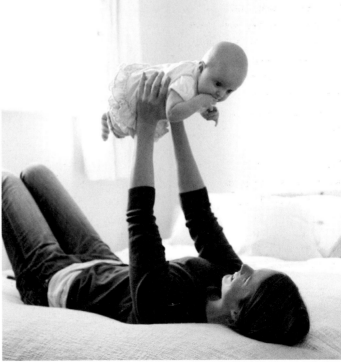

Toddler-lifting

Some toddlers weigh 13kg or more and require lifting many times during the day. This may be physically demanding, but it also provides you with the ideal means of working out and toning your body. Guidelines for lifting young children include using a half-kneeling lift from the floor. In this position, one knee is on the ground and the other leg is bent while you hold the child close to your centre and use your legs to push to a standing position without turning or twisting. When lifting a toddler from above your head, reverse the process and use the half-kneel position to lower your child.

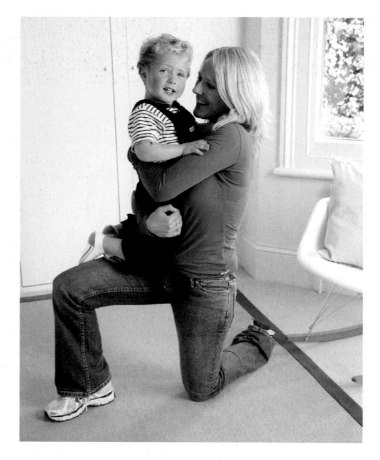

did you know?

Boogieing with (or without) the kids is a great way to burn more calories than you might imagine. Many types of dance are quite strenuous which makes them good for the heart and cardiovascular system. Even more sedate dances are equivalent to a 3mph walk, but something energetic like the quickstep, tango or jive will be more akin to a proper gym or aerobics session. When you dance, you engage your core muscles in the centre of your body around the trunk and lower back. At the same time, dancing uses the inter-scapular muscles (between the shoulder blades) so that the middle back opens up.

- An average 60kg adult will burn 150 calories after just half an hour of vigorous dancing. You will also find that you look longer and leaner the more frequently you dance. This is because the activity lengthens the distance from the hips to the pelvis which becomes crunched when you spend too long sitting down.

For most new mothers a lack of time, energy and childcare arrangements mean that baby bulges can persist for months after giving birth. However, help is at hand in the form of the latest fitness craze targeted at mums – buggy workouts – for which you needn't worry about finding a crèche because baby comes too! In America, the rise in popularity of buggy workouts has been meteoric – wherever you go, be it the park, a shopping mall, the beach or out on the street, you'll see brigades of mothers lunging and pushing their way to fitness. The best thing about it is that both mother and baby get to enjoy it. My son, Frankie, loves nothing better than for me to 'run' him to nursery in his jogging buggy; he chuckles and sings for the entire route and I get a great workout to boot!

Benefits for mind and body

Buggy-walking sessions are emotionally as well as physically beneficial to new mothers – a fact that has been documented by Australian researchers. Among women diagnosed with post-natal depression, the 20 who completed a 12 week buggy exercise session showed fewer symptoms than those in a sedentary mother-and-baby group. The researchers concluded that the sociability of buggy-walking (women went either with a friend or took part in a class), combined with the aerobic activity's ability to raise levels of the feel-good hormones, endorphins, produced the effects.

However, most women are first attracted to buggy workouts for the reshaping benefits. By alternating spurts of fast and slow walking you can vary the intensity of the workout and get fitter much more quickly.

Getting started

Classes are a good idea to get used to pushchair exercises, but they are not essential. Most follow the same format: for roughly an hour an instructor leads the way in a lung-busting stroll that forms the aerobic base of the workout with intermittent breaks to perform strengthening and toning moves. If you can't find a class, simply use the workout over the next few pages as a guideline.

Equipment required to start 'strollercising' is minimal. A pair of running or walking shoes, a tracksuit and a supportive sports bra (especially if you are breastfeeding) are the basics.

While any reasonably sturdy but lightweight buggy will suffice on tarmac and concrete surfaces, a more specialist design is a worthwhile investment if you plan to go off-road frequently or if you plan to run rather than walk with your child. Check that the handlebars are at a comfortable height and that the wheels are not positioned in a way that they trip you up. Ideally they should be easy to manoeuvre but also have some suspension to keep the baby comfortable. Buggies with added traction tyres and bigger wheels are ideal for those who get hooked. In America, strollercisers often progress to become stroller-runners, completing road races and fun runs while pushing their offspring.

Buggy sprints

Run fast with your buggy for 20 metres, preferably along a straight path in a park. Slow down to a jog or walk.

Repeat 5 times.

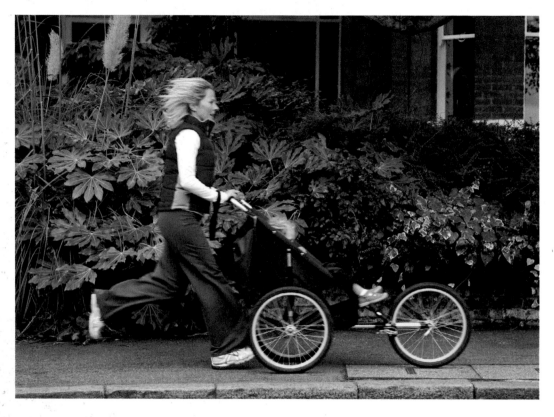

Buggy-ing

Start with a 15-minute power walk. You are working hard enough if you start to get a little sweaty and breathless.

Repeat this power walk for a few minutes between each exercise and for 10 minutes at the end.

Buggy-facing dips

Find a bench or a wall and position baby in the buggy facing you.

1 Place your hands on the bench and walk your legs out in front of you.

2 Lower yourself down towards the ground then raise yourself back up. You should feel this in the back of your arms.

Repeat 10 times.

Buggy lunges

You can do this exercise while walking or standing.

1 Holding onto the buggy, step forwards with your right leg.

2 Drop your bottom straight down until your right leg is at right angles to the floor.

3 Lift your bottom slowly back up until you are back in an upright position.

Repeat 15 times on alternate legs.

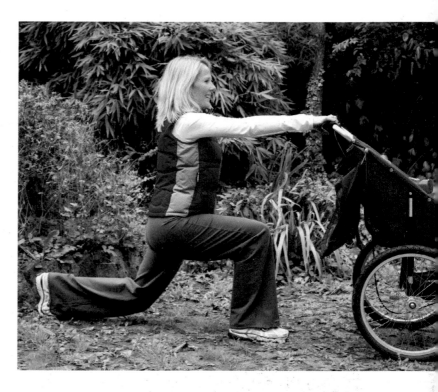

Buggy squats

1 Hold onto the buggy and from a standing position lower your bottom to a 90-degree angle as if you are sitting in a chair.

2 Hold for a second and return to a standing position, keeping your hands on the buggy for support only, not to pull yourself up.

Repeat 20 times.

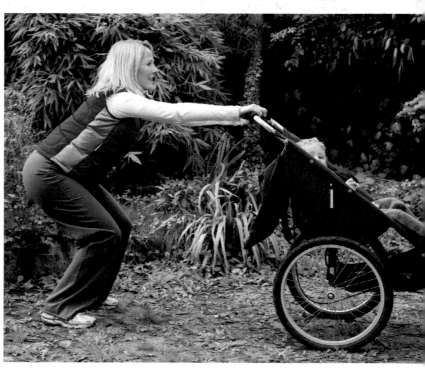

park workouts

Park circuits are a huge fitness trend in London and New York where organised classes take members through a range of gut-busting exercises using park benches, trees and walls as fitness tools. So, the next time you visit the park with your children, why not stage your own mini park Olympics. Set out a circuit that you can do as they play or get them to join in too.

Bench dips

These are great for toning the biceps muscles in the arms and for toning your upper body.

1 Find a bench and sit down with your feet flat on the ground. Inch forwards until your bottom and hands are on the edge of the seat. Your feet should remain flat on the floor and your legs should be bent at right angles.

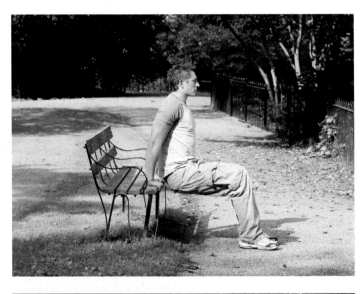

2 From here, slowly lower your body towards the ground, keeping your back as close to the bench as you can without touching it. Drop down until your upper arms are parallel with the ground. Slowly bring yourself back up again.

Perform 10 dips, rest and then stretch your arms for 30 seconds before repeating 3 times.

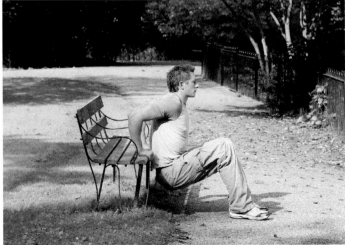

Bench crunches

You will need a bench or low wall for this exercise.

1 Sit on the ground facing the front of the bench, then lie down so that your back is on the floor and lift your legs on to the seat of the bench.

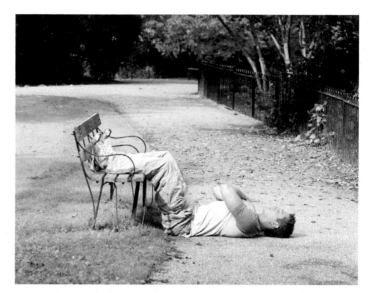

2 Shuffle forwards a little so that your thighs are at right angles to your calves. Cross your hands over your chest and contract your abdominal muscles as you curl upwards. Slowly roll back down.

Repeat 8–10 times, maintaining a rhythmic movement throughout.

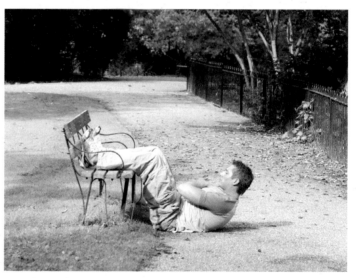

Piggy backs

Piggy backs are the height of fun, but they are also one of the best ways to develop all-over body strength. The important thing is to carry someone who weighs less or the same as you – so while you can piggy back your children around, you will need to hitch a lift from another adult. Try staging piggy-back races in the park, possibly including obstacles such as running around trees.

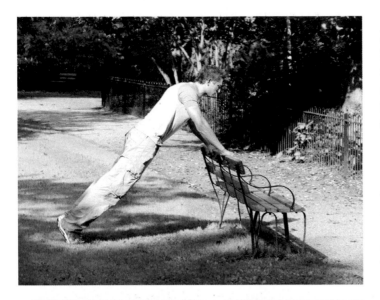

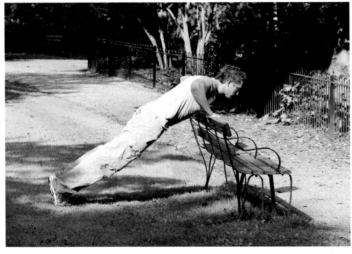

Bench push-ups

Push-ups are great for toning the upper body and for strengthening the pectoral muscles that give women the appearance of a pert bust.

1 Stand facing the back of a bench and place your hands shoulder-width apart on the seat back. Move a couple of feet backwards until your body forms a straight diagonal line from your feet to your head. Keep your bottom tucked in.

2 Slowly bend your arms so that you lower your chest towards the bench. Hold for a couple of seconds and then push back up until your arms are straight again.

Repeat 12 times without stopping if you can. If that is too much of a struggle, repeat 6 times, take a 20-second rest and then do 6 more.

Shuttle runs

Shuttle runs are a great way to develop cardiovascular fitness and speed endurance – footballers do a lot of them in training.

Find two trees that are about 10–15m apart. If this isn't possible just mark the distance by placing a bag or jumper on the ground. Run as fast as you can between the two markers, then turn swiftly, making sure you don't slow to a halt, and run back again. Do 6 sprints, then take a breather before doing 6 more.

As you get fitter try experimenting by hopping, bunny-jumping or side-stepping between the markers. The variety will take your muscles by surprise.

Hill marches

Walking uphill strengthens your cardiovascular system and it also burns about one-third more calories than walking on flat ground.

Find a gentle slope – around 50–80 metres in length – and march up to the top as fast as you can. Your feet should work from heel to toe and your weight should fall slightly forwards so you can push off your toes. Bend your arms and keep your elbows close to your body. Swing your arms from the shoulders, raising them towards your chest so that they are in line with your hips. Breathe normally at all times.

Perform 5 hill marches in a session, each followed by a gentler walk back down, but no stopping.

As you get fitter, you can practise swinging your arms in time with your legs and increasing your speed. Take short strides and remember to breathe rhythmically.

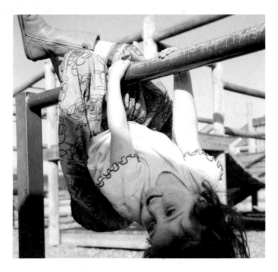

Playground fitness

Get into the park playground and climb and swing on the equipment with your children. This really is a workout in itself and will challenge all the muscles in the body. Plus, it is great fun.

work it out

Guzzling **a burger** when you are famished may stave off your hunger pangs for a while, but what will it do to your waistline? An average-sized burger from a fast-food chain contains 492 calories and a whopping 23g of fat. That total rises as you pile on mayonnaise or cheese and throw in a portion of fries. To negate the effects of your binge you would have to do one of the following:

- pack boxes for a house move for 1 hour and 15 minutes
- do 1 hour and 30 minutes of drilling with a power drill
- push someone in a wheelchair or push a wheelbarrow full of heavy materials for 61 minutes
- deal with uncooperative children for 1 hour and 20 minutes – chasing, dressing and lifting them into a car seat, etc.
- do 1 hour and 38 minutes of unloading a washing machine and hanging the clothes out on the line
- play non-stop hopscotch with the kids for 70 minutes.

Having children should not be an excuse to give up on the sexual side of your relationship. Yes, kids might leave you exhausted, but having regular romps with your partner can leave you revitalised and re-energised enough to cope with anything life throws at you. It also constitutes a workout that can get you feeling fit and help to ward off a range of illnesses and minor complaints.

In exercise – or sexercise – terms, sex uses every muscle in the body while burning up to 200 calories an hour in a very enjoyable workout. The pulse rate of a sexually excited person increases from 70 to 150 beats a minute and just one love-in burns off the same number of calories as running on a treadmill for 15 minutes. Daily sex can also whittle away 500g of your weight per week.

But the effects extend far beyond the bedroom. Prior to an orgasm, the brain emits a dose of the hormone oxytocin which results in the production of sedative endorphins – natural derivatives of morphine. Therefore, sex is considered a tremendous painkiller. Many people with joint problems such as arthritis find that they feel better 45 minutes to 3 hours after intercourse because of these effects. One study found that, for women and men, orgasms eased migraines faster than any medicine.

Sex can also ward off a bout of the sniffles. Psychologists have found that people who have sex once or twice a week have levels of immunoglobulin A (IgA) – a powerful antibody that boosts the immune system – up to a third higher than their less sexually active counterparts. Scientists have also found that an active sex life may lower the risk of developing cancer and strokes.

According to one British study, sexercise can even lower the risk of heart attacks and help you to live longer. Having sex lowered blood pressure for up to a week. Precisely why this happens is unknown, but it could be that intercourse stimulates a variety of nerves which are directly involved in soothing and calming the brain and body.

Exercise and sex are inextricably linked. One study showed that people with active sex lives tend to exercise more often and have better eating habits than others. To make your regular romp even more worthwhile, try the following sexercise workout.

Give it some oomph

As everyone knows, women take longer than men to reach an orgasm. To make sure you both get a cardiovascular workout, swap the lead so that male and female partners alternately do the most work. And put some oomph into your love-making. Really make your partner sweat.

Work your butt

Your bottom is not there just to appeal to the opposite sex. Its muscles perform a vital function during the thrusting phase of sex. In fact, the thrust has the same benefits as squatting at the gym when it comes to toning the butt and legs, so work as hard as you can.

Flatten your stomach

Having intercourse in the missionary position can be hard work for the partner on top, but it will help to tone their tummy in the process. Exercise scientists claim the practice of holding your abdominal muscles in tightly as you move up and down (which is similar to something called the 'plank' position in Pilates) is a great way to work the core musculature, essential for avoiding back pain and improving posture as well as for getting rid of a pot belly.

Clench your kegels

No, this is not some weird sex toy, but a group of muscles called the pubococcygeal muscles that strengthen the walls of the vagina, making childbirth easier, incontinence less likely and orgasms more intense. To locate your kegels (as these muscles are more commonly known), try stopping your flow of urine mid-stream. Clenching the kegel muscles for 5–8 seconds several times a day and during love-making can have profound health effects.

Bend and stretch

Become more flexible during love-making by trying as many different positions in as many different places as possible. Improved flexibility means a better range of movement around the body's joints which results in a lower risk of injury. And being as bendy as a ballerina means you can also be more creative between the sheets.

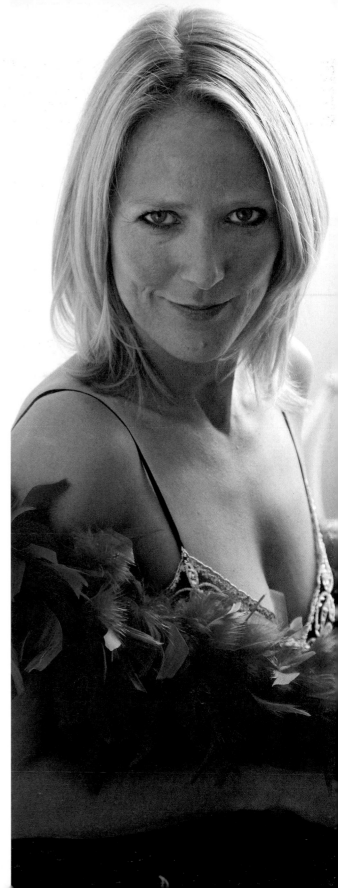

chapter seven

How did you stay fit as a child? If you grew up in the 1960s, 70s or 80s the chances are that fitness and fatness never even entered your vocabulary until you became an adult because you were far too busy playing outside and running around. How our lives have changed. There are many worrying statistics published about children and the threats to young lives today, but none so disturbing, perhaps, as those that show how this 'cotton wool' generation is being protected to such an extent that they are no longer being allowed the freedom to play.

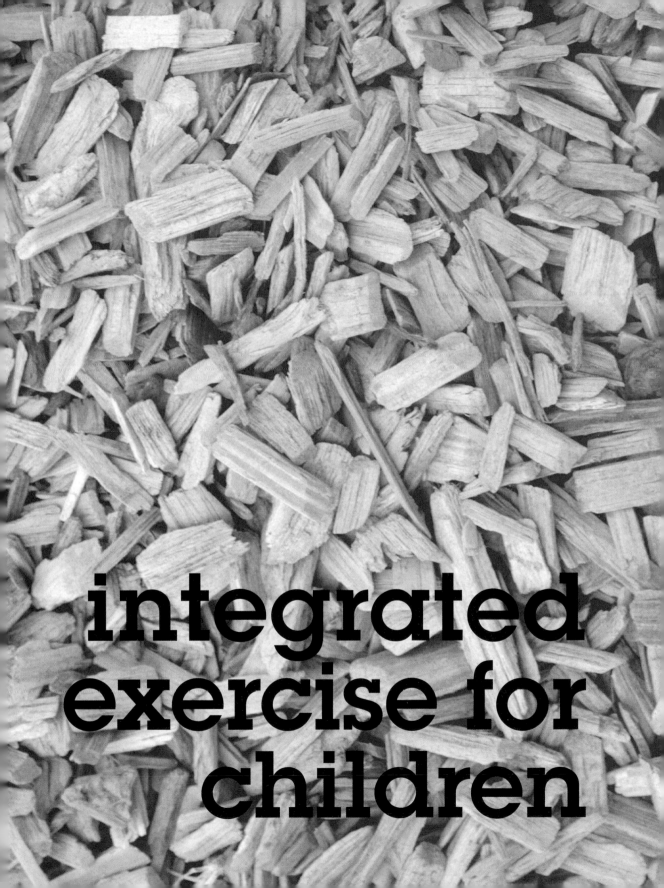

integrated exercise for children

a healthier childhood

Too many parents now deny their children the kind of unsupervised outdoor play that they themselves enjoyed, because of fears for their safety. A report by the Children's Society in the UK showed that almost half of 1,148 adults questioned said they believed children should not be allowed out with friends until they were fourteen, but most said they had been allowed out without supervision aged ten or younger.

Undoubtedly, this lack of childhood activity is fuelling a rise in obesity among the toddler-to-teen age groups. One report in the medical journal the *Lancet* showed that today's youngsters are the first in history to be less healthy than their parents and almost one-third of Britain's children aged two to eleven are overweight or obese. It is a picture that is pretty much the same throughout the Western world.

But other factors beyond weight are being affected. Physical activity helps to develop so many different skills as well as psychological and emotional strengths that they are almost too numerous to mention. A few of the main advantages are listed below, but ultimately the most important things you can hope to bring to your child's life by encouraging them to be more active are good health, fun and enjoyment. Isn't that what childhood is supposed to be about?

work it out

According to the British Heart Foundation's latest campaign, one half of British children eat a **packet of crisps** a day. Since a small bag (28g) of ready salted crisps contains around 132 calories and 6.2g of fat, the BHF says that such snacking habits means crisp guzzlers consume almost 5 litres of cooking oil a year. To work off the calories in one bag of crisps, you would need to do one of the following:

- stretch or do light yoga for 1 hour
- go in-line skating for 27 minutes
- play table tennis for 25 minutes
- go fishing and walk along the riverbank for 30 minutes
- spend 33 minutes unloading your supermarket shopping and putting it away
- sand wooden floors with a power sander for 24 minutes
- skip with a rope for 18 minutes.

five reasons to get your kids active

1 Activity has positive effects not only on a child's physical development, but on their academic and social development too. Surveys show that children who are regularly active will achieve higher grades in school and have better behaviour records.

2 A study by researchers at Oxford University demonstrated that young people who take part in regular physical activity have improved social skills and self-esteem.

3 Children who are active are more likely to become active adults and less likely to become obese or dangerously overweight. In other words, instil the habit now and it might last for a lifetime.

4 Play and physical activity are among the best ways to develop a child's creativity and imagination. Making mud pies, building dens, making up games and staging mini plays/sports days in the garden do more to fire their enthusiasm and imagination than any pre-organised or commercial activity.

5 Children who play at school are less likely to be bullied. One study found that introducing more old-fashioned playground games such as skipping, hopscotch and hula hoops led to a more sociable atmosphere and less bullying.

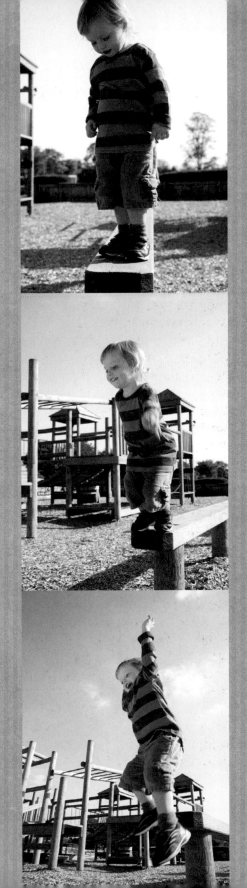

how much activity do children need?

How long is a piece of string? Left to their own devices, children are instinctively good judges of how much (or how little) they need to play, sleep and eat. However, health organisations do set suggestions for minimum levels of play and activity that are needed for a child to ward off obesity and stay healthy.

In the UK, no specific guidelines are set for children under the age of six, but they are likely to be in line with those set by the American Academy of Pediatrics (AAP) which recommends only 15 minutes of 'structured activity' – i.e. specific games such as football, throwing a ball or swimming – for the under-fives.

Beyond that age, all 5-to-18 year olds should participate in an absolute minimum of an hour of moderate-intensity activity every day at school or elsewhere. At least twice a week this should include activities to improve bone health, muscle strength and flexibility such as those involving running, climbing, cycling or any sport. School should play a vital role in introducing the benefits and enjoyment of physical activity to your child.

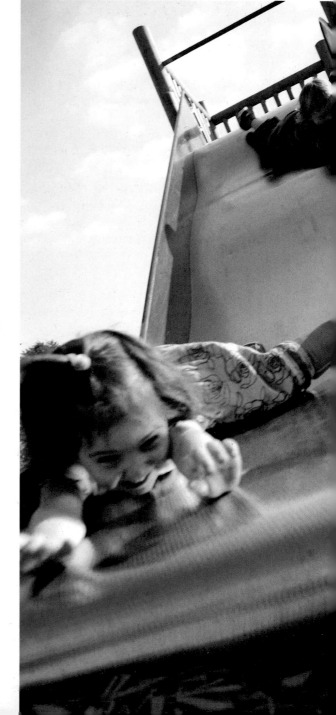

playground games to introduce to your children

Why not relive your own childhood by reintroducing some traditional playground games to your children?

Bulldog

A game for up to fifteen players in which they race to see who is in the middle and this person has to tag people trying to get past them. If you get tagged you join the person in the middle in trying to tag others. The game ends when everyone is in the middle. Last one in starts in the centre for the next game.

Hide and seek

One person is 'it' and they are the seeker who will look for the other players. The person who is 'it' covers their eyes or looks away and counts to an agreed number while the rest of the players hide. When the counting is finished, 'it' says, 'Coming, ready or not' and runs to find everyone. The last player to be found is the winner.

French skipping

This game helps to develop precision jumping skills and supreme concentration. To play you need a long piece of knicker elastic around 5mm wide. A good length would be about 3 metres. A minimum of three players is needed, two of whom stand inside the loop, stretching it relatively taut around their ankles, while the remaining player performs a series of jumping moves landing in specific agreed positions in relation to the elastic. For example:

both feet under the elastic; both feet on top of the elastic; one on top, one under; and so on. After a full round of all the jumps has been completed, the height of the elastic is raised to 'kneesies', then 'thighsies', 'waistsies' and then the real challenge, which is 'chestsies'. If the player fails to execute the correct jump their turn is over and play passes to the next person.

Ultimate frisbee

A competitive version of this game is played by adults. But for the playground version, you will need one frisbee and a relatively flat piece of land. There are two teams, each with a minimum of two players. Each team has a 'goal' area and the point of the game is to get the frisbee into your goal area. At the start of the game, teams start opposite their goal area and a member of one team throws the frisbee towards the middle. Both teams can then rush in and whoever gets to it first/catches it starts play, which involves simply passing the frisbee back and forth among the team to try to make it to the goal area. After this there are a few rules. First, the person who has the frisbee cannot move more than three steps without passing it. Second, they may not hold on to it for more than 10 seconds. Breaking these rules means that the other team gets the frisbee. When passing the frisbee, the other team may intercept by either catching or moving it in any way so that the other team cannot catch it and that means that they can now play the frisbee. Also, if the frisbee is dropped (or not caught) it automatically switches teams. Once one team gets their frisbee to their goal area, they have a point. The teams move to their respective ends of the field and the team that did not get the last point gets to throw in the frisbee. This goes on until exhaustion.

ten great ways to get your kids moving

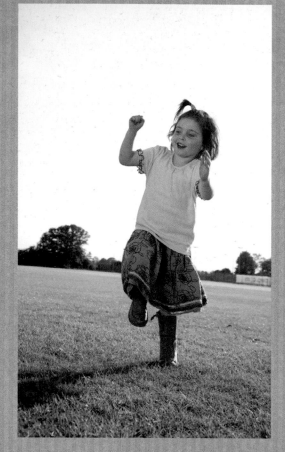

1 **Get down on the floor:** What could be more simple than just sitting on the floor to play with your children? One of the biggest mistakes parents make is to think that any activity has to be a really complex, packaged programme. And it's no good thinking you can sit your child in front of the TV then compensate by paying for them to go to a gym class. The key is just to get your children moving as a way of life and make sure it's fun. Just be inventive.

2 **Turn off the TV:** The American Academy of Pediatrics committee on sports medicine and fitness recommends no TV for children under the age of two and no more than 2 hours daily of total screen time (i.e. TV, computer, videogames) for older children.

3 **Be a good role model:** Studies have found that children whose parents exercise are more likely to do so themselves. The more active you are, the more likely your children are to follow suit.

4 **Go to the park:** For sheer variety of physical challenges there is not much that tops the average park playground with its swings, climbing frames, roundabouts and see-saws. Playing for an hour in a park will help to develop everything from balance to spatial awareness and from muscle strength to self-confidence. Let them play themselves to exhaustion.

5 **Play hopping and jumping games:** Hopping and jumping are great ways to improve leg strength and power. They also help to stimulate bone growth which is most prolific during childhood and early teens. Most top sports people use hopping in their training regimes. Stage a mini competition to see who can perform the fewest hops over a 30-metre course. Repeat using bunny hops (i.e. double-footed jumps). And don't forget the classic playground game of hopscotch: hopping on one foot, then jumping on both across a series of chalked boxes develops explosive muscle power and is a tremendous bone builder.

6 **Leapfrog to fitness:** This is a great way for your child to develop upper-body strength. Pushing off a partner's back to perform the leapfrog is energetic and recruits all the muscles in the arms, chest and back. But even the bending over phase is hard work as they must support the body weight of a partner.

7 **Try pogo sticking:** This activity is very much in vogue with adults in America where whole fitness classes are devoted entirely to it. Kinesiologists at Kansas State University suggest it is a low-impact route to fitness and an alternative to skipping. Their tests showed that hopping on a pogo stick caused the rapid leg-muscle contractions needed to build muscle tone, but that it was much less stressful to the joints than other activities.

8 **Balance and bounce on space hoppers:** Of course, adults now have their own version of the bright orange space hopper in the form of the Swiss balls used to perform abdominal and other exercises. But they are nowhere near as much fun as these toys. Bouncing around on a space hopper requires the use of leg, bottom and tummy muscles.

9 **Go for the standing long, triple and high jumps:** Although these are most closely related to track and field, the explosive power they require is crucial in most sports and activities. From a standing position, mark and measure the distance your child can jump vertically, horizontally or with a hop, step and then a jump. Keep a record and let them try to improve their distance periodically.

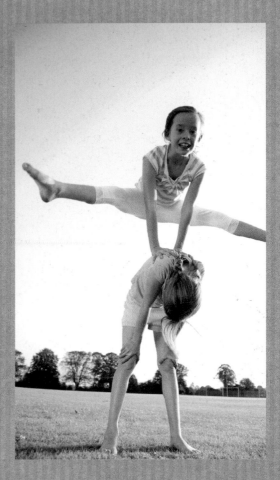

10 **Encourage a competitive spirit:** Sport is defined by its element of competition and learning to win and lose are vital components when it comes to fostering a child's enjoyment of sport. However, that doesn't mean your children have to join high-pressured sports clubs or get expert coaching from a very young age. Make competition fun. Stage mini races in the garden and get children to have competitions as to how high they can jump, how far they can run from one point to the next, or how far they can throw a Frisbee. Be imaginative.

tree-climbing

Climbing up (and falling out) of trees was once as much a part of childhood as comics and sweets. Not any more. According to a report by the UK's Royal Society for the Prevention of Accidents (RoSPA), today's children are more likely to suffer repetitive strain injuries (RSI) from overusing computer games than from tumbling out of a tree and figures from UK hospitals back this up.

This is worrying in terms of inactivity levels – tree climbing is incredibly energetic and moving from branch to branch calls on all the body's muscles – but also in terms of a child's preparation for life. Experiencing a small injury from an accident such as falling out of a tree teaches children about risk. Adult life is inherently risky. Without the lessons previously learned in childhood, how are today's youngsters going to cope tomorrow?

strange but true

For parents who are cautious about letting their children play in trees, expert help is at hand. An organisation called Tree Climbers International offers tuition courses on how to climb trees safely at over 50,000 sites both in the USA and in Europe. Children can also experience tree camping on their courses – childhood as it should be.

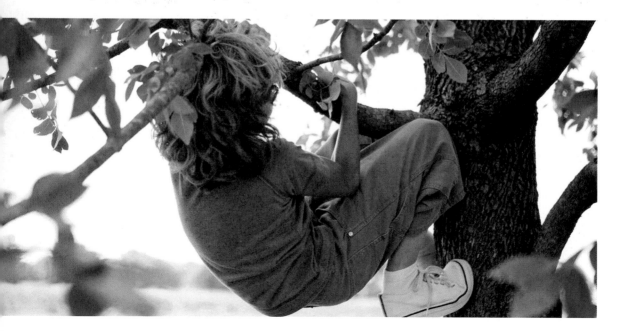

can computer games be active?

What sets the newest wave of computer games apart is that they allow players to mimic the physical aspects of a sport via a hand-held remote-control unit that communicates wirelessly with a sensor sitting on the television. Unlike other games that require little more activity than the repetitive pressing of thumbs and fingers on a console, when using these new interactive sports games, players must move, jump even – backwards, forwards, sideways and upwards – to get the highest scores.

In many ways, then, it seems the perfect compromise – yes, it's a computer game, but it is also, perhaps, a solution in part, to the obesity epidemic. At least that is what the manufacturers would have a generation of parents anxious about the inactive lifestyles of their children believe. But are they a substitute for the real thing and do they get children active enough to benefit their health?

Results of a study at John Moore's University in England provided promising statistics about one active computer game's ability to burn calories. It found that, in theory, regular use could shift 12kg in weight a year. Sounds impressive, but closer inspection of the research (which was part-funded by a computer game's marketing company), reveals the figures were based on an average 12.2 hours of 'gaming' a week by 13–15 year olds. So, while the game burned 40 per cent more calories than using a traditional console (i.e. while sitting on the sofa), it was never going to be as effective as getting out and playing the real thing, the scientists admitted. In my opinion, the bottom line is that these are still computer games. A television set is still the focus and, in that respect, they still promote a slothful, inactive lifestyle.

skipping

Skipping is undergoing something of a revival in the school playground which is great news for the health and fitness levels of children. This simple activity builds bones, burns fat and improves leg strength as well as any other.

Many teachers now use skipping in PE classes as a form of 'brain gym' for pupils, to refocus their attention and get rid of pent-up tensions. Techniques like the Double Dutch (in which two ropes rotate in egg-beater motion around one to two skippers) are incredibly demanding. And there are also moves like crossovers, pretzels and wing-dings which challenge you in many different ways. Elite skippers rarely just jump over the rope; rather they incorporate up to 200 different kinds of 'manouevres' and, in competitions, can perform push-ups, cartwheels and handstands while skipping over a rope spinning at 200 rpm.

Body benefits

The US National Institute of Health claims that skipping (or jump-roping) burns more calories than any other popular exercise except for fast running. Ten minutes of moderate skipping, they say, will burn 70 calories; if you are extremely energetic, you can eliminate 110 calories during the same time. Experienced skippers can burn up to 1300 calories in an hour of vigorous rope activity.

As part of its Jump Rope for Heart campaign, the British Heart Foundation offers free skipping workshops for teachers, designed to link to the national curriculum, highlighting how this form of exercise can help to combat the obesity problem among schoolchildren.

Getting started

Beyond its body-changing capabilities, the obvious attractions of skipping are that it is cheap and portable – invest a few pounds in a rope and you have a ready-made workout wherever you go. Avoid traditional, woven rope as it's heavy (even more so when wet) and slow to turn, making many of the moves more difficult. Ball bearings and jump counters also add unnecessary weight and make the ropes more cumbersome. The best bet is a lightweight, flexible plastic or leather gymnastic speed rope.

To make sure that the rope is the correct length for your child's height, stand them on the middle of the rope and let them pull the handles upwards until the rope is taut. The handles should line up with their shoulder blades – if they come up higher, cut a few inches of rope off one end, or tie it, until the length is correct.

> ### did you know?
> Children should be encouraged to set themselves mini goals, such as simply wanting to get faster: to break the world speed skipping record they would need to exceed 188 jumps in 30 seconds!

Skipping safely

Children should **take it slowly**, starting with a 1:3 skipping:rest ratio, so if they skip for 5 minutes they then rest for 15 and build up slowly.

Make sure the children (and you) are **wearing appropriate shoes,** such as cross-trainers or aerobic shoes, as these provide appropriate stability and cushioning under the forefoot.

Choose a well-lit area, preferably with a springy wooden floor or a carpeted surface, or put a thin, non-slip exercise mat down first.

Watch for posture. Knees and ankles should be bent and the torso straight when jumping. Arms should be by the skipper's side, with the rope turning from the wrists and forearms.

Before skipping, make sure your children do 5 minutes of gentle cardiovascular exercise, such as walking or marching. Then they should gently stretch all the major muscle groups. Remember they should also cool down, bringing the heart rate down gently at the end of a session. Stretches should be repeated.

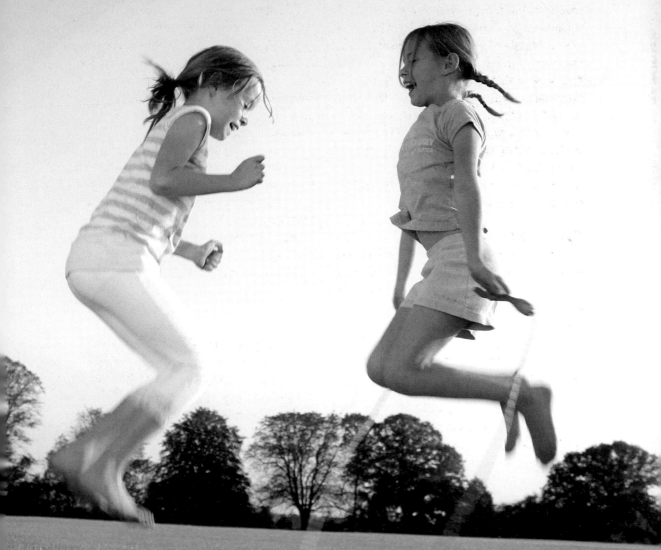

hooping

The hula hoop is currently enjoying something of a resurgence in popularity, not among children, but adults, who have discovered the hoop's ability to tone the waist and burn calories. For children however, hooping is something that deserves to grace playgrounds once again.

Body benefits

Not only is it great fun, but vigorous hooping can leave kids more than a little breathless. The traditional hooping movement – where the hoop is rotated around hips and waist using circular movements of the hips and trunk – recruits all the major muscles. Although the main movement is in the midriff, the legs also feed into the circling rhythm and work hard to keep the body steady. Because it uses upper and lower body (the arms are held up to stabilise the body) it helps to get the heart beating a little faster.

And there is plenty more you can do with a hula hoop. Experienced hoopers use it to tone their entire bodies, spiraling it around their ankles, wrists, neck and arms. They even practise 'tush whirls' which involve bending over at the waist so that the chest is parallel to the floor and circling the hoop around their bottom.

did you know?

Trainers with wheels in the heels have captured a loyal following largely among children aged six to fourteen. But are they a good way for kids to integrate exercise? A top ten of the world's worst toys of 2006 saw wheeled trainers take top spot amid claims that they put users at risk of head and spinal injuries as well as postural and muscular complaints. With the wheel situated in the heel of the shoe, the dynamics of walking are changed in wearers of wheeled shoes, claim experts. Physiotherapists say they also adversely affect the way children walk: normally, our heel strikes the ground first when we walk, but the wheels prevent that and so a child is forced to alter their technique or gait accordingly. Instead they have to lift their knees, a bit like a horse, which is not a good thing at such a young age. In the long term, it could stress ill-prepared parts of the body and cause overuse injuries. However, they're not all bad news — on the positive side, according to some experts, heeling may help a little with spatial awareness and balance and will contribute towards the recommended daily minimum of an hour of activity a day for children. It may also encourage them to take up ice- or roller-skating each of which is demanding in its own right.

Getting started

Choose a hoop with ball bearings for a smoother action (they will give a distinctive *shoop-shoop* sound as you twirl). Heavier, weighted hoops are available for adults who want to get fit as they hoop with the kids. Trials at the Cooper Institute for Human Performance and Nutrition Research in Dallas found that vigorous circling with a heavier hoop for about 8 minutes burns as many calories – about 110 – as running a 10-minute mile. Less strenuous hooping uses a similar amount of energy (85 calories) to that you would expend on a very slow mile-long jog.

Technique

Set the hoop against the small of your back and hold it so that it is parallel to the ground before you start to twirl. Keep your hands out and feet fairly close together so that you are well balanced and circle your hips in a small movement.

chapter eight

Going on holiday – or a business trip – and leaving your regular activity routine behind does not have to mean that a lardier version of you comes back two weeks later. In fact, choose the right activity and you may find you end up fitter and leaner than before.

integrated exercise for the traveller

on planes and trains

If you do travel by plane or train regularly, make sure you inject a little activity into your journey with these exercises:

- Squeeze a tennis ball with your hands until they're tired.

- Keep the balls of your feet on the floor and raise your legs using your calf muscles. To make it tougher, place some extra weight (a bag or laptop computer) on your knees. Repeat 15 times.

- To stretch your calf muscles, keep your heels firmly on the ground and lift your toes as high as possible. Hold for 5 seconds, and relax. Repeat 15 times.

- Place your hands on the armrests of your seat and lift both of your knees slowly towards your chin. Lower slowly and repeat 10 times.

- Keep your chin close to your throat and tilt your head forwards. Carefully roll your head from one shoulder to the other, but avoid rotating it backwards.

- Contract your gluteus (bottom) muscles as tightly as you can and hold for 20 seconds. These muscles are the biggest in the human body and need to be exercised too.

work it out

What could be more refreshing than **an ice cream** on a hot day? However, if you select a chocolate-covered ice lolly, you could be guzzling as many as 260 calories (139 of them from fat). To burn that off you'd need to do one of the following:

- 37 minutes of riding a pedalo
- 33 minutes of energetic play in a park – on swings, slides and climbing frames
- 34 minutes of ballet
- 32 minutes of arm cycling (i.e. using an arm-cycling machine with vigorous effort)
- 28 minutes of scuba diving.

- Get up and walk around at least once every hour. As you stroll about, alternate balancing yourself on the balls of your feet, then on your heels.

- With fingers interlaced and palms inverted, stretch your arms overhead, then twist your upper body to each side. This can be done seated or standing.

thirteen great ways to integrate exercise on holiday

Holidays are a time for relaxing and quiet reflection, but they can also be a great time to integrate new and unusual activities into your day. Here's how to ensure you keep active as well as have fun during your vacation:

1 Go for a swim: Swimming is great for the injury-prone as the water acts as a giant cushion to protect your joints. It is also generally regarded as the best all-round fitness activity as it works all of the body's major muscle groups and has an aerobic effect. Different strokes work different muscle groups, so incorporating backstroke, butterfly, breaststroke and front crawl means you will cover the range. Swimming front crawl in an indoor pool will burn around 300 calories in half an hour; take to the sea, however, and you burn extra calories as your body encounters waves, currents and the elements.

2 Hire a jet ski: These petrol-engined, water-propelled speed merchants are generically known as personal water craft (PWCs), jet ski being the trade name. Jet skiing is not as physically demanding as many water sports (although some effort is required in the upper body for steering and manoeuvring), but the adrenaline buzz they provide is second to none. Some models can reach speeds of up to 70mph but many launch sites set speed limits much lower than this.

3 Play beach volleyball: This sport, which hit the Olympic scene in 1996, has gained a reputation as one of the most glamorous to watch thanks to the fact that elite female competitors tend to be tanned, blonde and Amazonian in physique, wearing the teeniest bikini briefs possible. The object of the game is to get the ball over the net and into the opponents' side of the court. This inevitably involves jumping and sprinting which develop explosive power and work muscles in the legs and bottom. Shoulders and the upper body are also tested, so it is little wonder the pros are models of lean perfection.

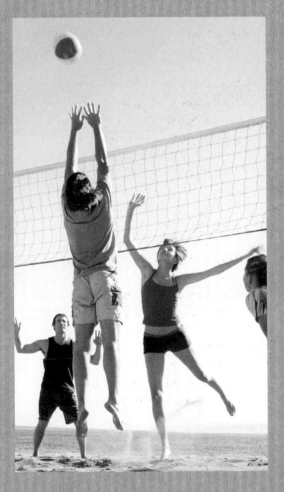

4 **Go beach-walking ...** Don't just vegetate on your sun lounger. Walking even short distances barefoot on soft sand – the type found higher up on beaches – will do you good as it requires you to use more energy than you would walking on concrete or Tarmac. Every time your foot hits the ground it creates a small depression so that the leg muscles must work harder to push upwards and forwards for the next step. Experts also suggest shortening your stride for a more even-footed landing and keeping your weight balanced to avoid sinking in.

The fact that sand is softer than pavement also means less stress to the joints. If you prefer running to walking, stick to the wet, firm-packed sand near the shoreline at low tide because the surface is flatter and less punishing on the body. Avoid running on the shore's slopes, which can cause imbalances and strain in the knees, calves and ankles.

5 **... or sea-walking** Some Florida gyms are offering fitness classes in sea-walking and it is little wonder. Next time you are walking along the beach, try walking in the water up to your ankles. The combination of resistance from both the water and the sand will give you a great workout. Walking in the ocean against the current will also give you a good lower-body workout.

6 **Power-walk in the pool:** Water acts as a giant cushion for the body and is much kinder to joints and tendons than tarmac and other surfaces. The deeper you wade into a pool, the lighter your body becomes. American research has shown that waist-deep water reduces the pressure on joints by 50 per cent and chest-deep by 75 per cent, but if you work out in water up to neck level, as with aqua-running, your body weight is effectively reduced by as much as 90 per cent. If you decide you like the activity, consider buying a pair of aqua trainers designed to protect your feet from abrasions and to provide added resistance of up to 30 per cent so that you work even harder. Pools are built for swimming so their bottoms can be rough and your feet will probably feel it at the end of a workout. Wade in at waist level and you could burn 270 calories in half an hour.

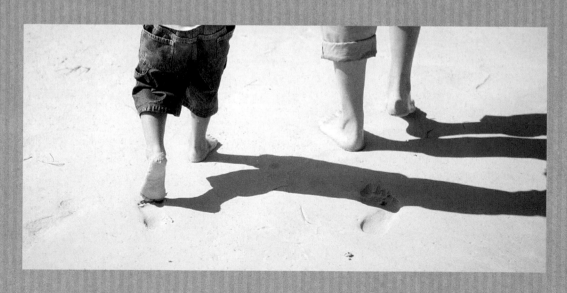

7 **Learn to windsurf:** Compared with other water sports, windsurfing is easier (and cheaper) to learn. Mastering it is dependent more on good technical skill than brute strength which means that women and children are not at a disadvantage; improved equipment (such as lighter weight boards) also makes it easier to manage in the water. Staying upright requires you to engage all the major muscle groups – as does hauling yourself back on board when you fall off!

8 **Hire a pedalo:** Using pedal power to propel the craft through the water means that most of the major muscles will be worked in the legs and buttocks. The faster you pedal and the stronger the wind against you, the more calories you will burn (up to 400 an hour). Your heart and lungs will benefit if you keep going long enough and do it regularly.

9 **Play beach bat and ball:** A beach variation on tennis, this offers a full-body workout involving an impressive number of muscle groups. The power for a shot is initiated from ground level – the strength for a great serve is provided by the push-off from the quadriceps in your thighs. Sharp twists and turns put the abdominals and upper body through a vigorous workout. Using the racket and hitting the ball exercises your arms and shoulders. Your forearms absorb the impact from the ball contact and your shoulders and upper arms are strengthened all over as they respond with various strokes from overhead to ground level.

10 **Try wakeboarding:** Wakeboarding is to waterskiing what snowboarding is to skiing – the younger, cooler version which uses one board not two. Proponents claim it is a fusion of snowboarding and surfing: the rider, whose feet are attached to the board with bindings, is towed by a boat. Steering is achieved by using board edges in much the same way as a snowboarder does. It requires a good level of all-round fitness and exceptional strength in the upper body as well as the legs to execute well.

11 **Get in a kayak:** The upper-body action which includes twisting as well as pushing and pulling with the arms, is one of the best ways to tone your midriff. Water provides resistance acting as a weight-training aid as you propel yourself forwards.

12 **Perform a pool workout:** Try a mini-aqua-aerobics session. Warm up with a swim. Then, in the shallow end, do 90 seconds each of walking lunges, squats, and leg lifts to the front side and back, holding on to the edge. For muscle endurance go to the deep end and tread water as long as you can for the finale. Tread just with your arms, then just with your legs, then with both together.

13 **Build a sandcastle:** Set yourself the task of building the biggest and best sandcastle on the beach. Scooping up armfuls of sand will work the biceps and triceps muscles in your arms. Complete your efforts by surrounding the castle with a moat and you will have completed a full-body workout.

hotel-room workout

Exercise is the best way to help you tune into different time zones, especially after a long-haul flight. Long periods of inactivity on a plane, combined with the dehydrated atmosphere of air travel can leave you feeling sluggish and lethargic when you land. While you don't have to jump into activity mode immediately when you arrive – although it is recommended you go for a walk when you can – try to do at least some of the exercises below while you are away.

These exercises don't call for a gym or any fancy equipment, yet they form some of the best moves around for different body parts. Try doing a circuit by performing one set of each exercise, and then starting again with the first. Or, challenge yourself to do three sets of a single exercise to really fatigue that muscle group, before moving on to the next.

Always start with a gentle warm-up of walking on the spot (or up some stairs) for 5 minutes.

Pert chest

Often overlooked by exercisers, the chest muscles are actually recruited for most of the things we do – from mowing the lawn to carrying shopping. Problems can arise when weak chest muscles (or pectorals) become tight and shortened as a result of being hunched over a desk or steering wheel for hours on end. To strengthen the pectoral and surrounding muscles, try the chest press.

1 Lie on the floor on your back, arms out to the sides, holding a bottle of water in each hand.

2 Bend your knees so that your feet are flat on the floor and press the hollow of your back into the floor.

3 Gradually raise both arms until your hands meet at the top. Slowly lower the water bottles back down until they are about 5cm off the ground.

Repeat 10 times.

Press-ups are also great for toning the chest (see page 142).

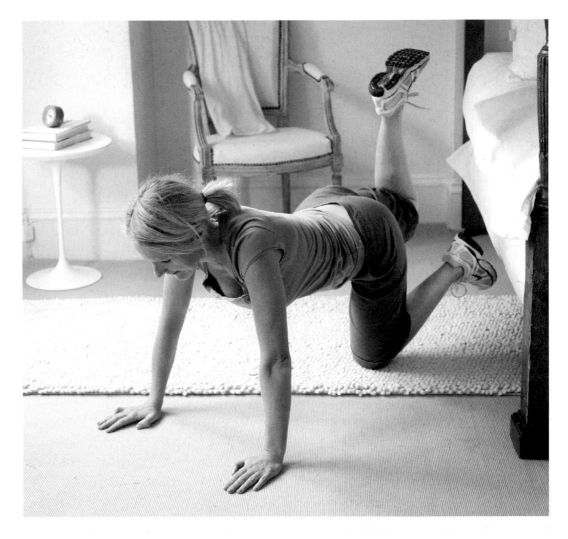

Bottom tightener

A pert bottom is the number-one concern for many people. An American study recorded and compared the levels of muscle activation in a number of different exercises in order to establish the best way to achieve buttocks of steel. Quadruped hip extensions came out top and here's how to do them:

1 On your hands and knees, contract your abdominals to stabilise your torso.

2 Lift one leg up, keeping the knee bent at 90 degrees, until the bottom of the foot is pointing towards the ceiling and the leg is lined up with the body.

Lower and repeat 10–15 times.

Add ankle weights to make the quadruped exercise more challenging and increase the repetitions as you get stronger.

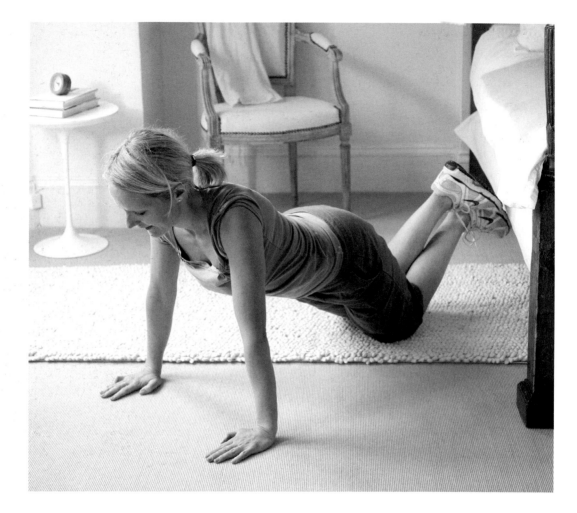

Arm toner

Sometimes the simplest exercises are the most effective and never more so than when it comes to the arms. Plain, old-fashioned press-ups are the best bet as they use the weight of the body to work the triceps, pectorals and deltoids (arm, chest and shoulder muscles). One study found that a programme of regular press-ups improved both strength and power in the arms and upper body. Start with half press-up (keeping your knees on the floor) and progress to the full press-up as you get stronger.

1 Lie face down on the floor, hands by your shoulders and knees bent. Press your palms into the floor, straightening your arms.

2 Keep your head, neck, back, and hips in line as you lift your body off the floor.

3 When your arms are almost fully extended, hold. Now slowly lower yourself back down, but just before you touch the floor, push back up again.

Repeat 10–20 times, progressively adding more repetitions until you can comfortably manage 30.

Back strengthener

Research has revealed that many conventional back-training practices, including stretching regimes and strength-training moves can actually make back pain worse. So what is the best exercise for back strength? Top of the list came the curl-up:

1 Lie flat on your back with one knee flexed.

2 Raise your head and shoulders off the floor

Repeat 10–15 times, alternating the bent leg mid-way through each set of repetitions.

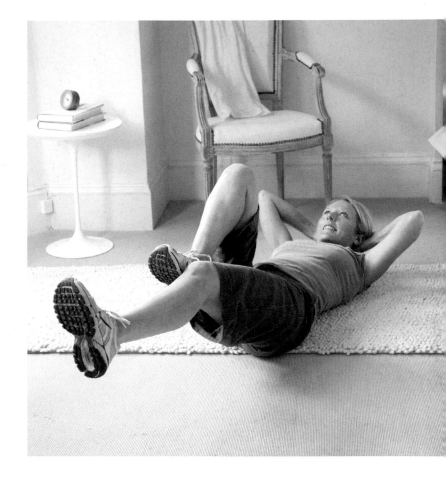

Leg lengthener

Another finding of the study to find the best bottom exercises (see page 141) was that lunges are among the best exercises for targeting the leg and gluteal muscles together. Here's how to do them.

1 Hold a bottle of water in each hand, standing tall with good posture.

2 Step forwards with your right foot, keeping your head up and spine neutral (i.e. neither bent nor taut).

3 Drop your left knee towards the floor by bending the knees, making sure to keep the front heel down and the knee directly over the centre of the foot.

4 Push down and forwards through your heel to return to the starting position.

Repeat on the other side, alternating for 8–12 repetitions on each side.

chapter nine

Having made the decision to integrate exercise into your lifestyle, the next essential step is to make sure your diet comes up to scratch. Eating should be straightforward – after all, food is just the fuel that we need to stay alive, no more, no less. But something so simple has become complicated to such an extent that very few people now feel confident in selecting a diet to suit their everyday needs.

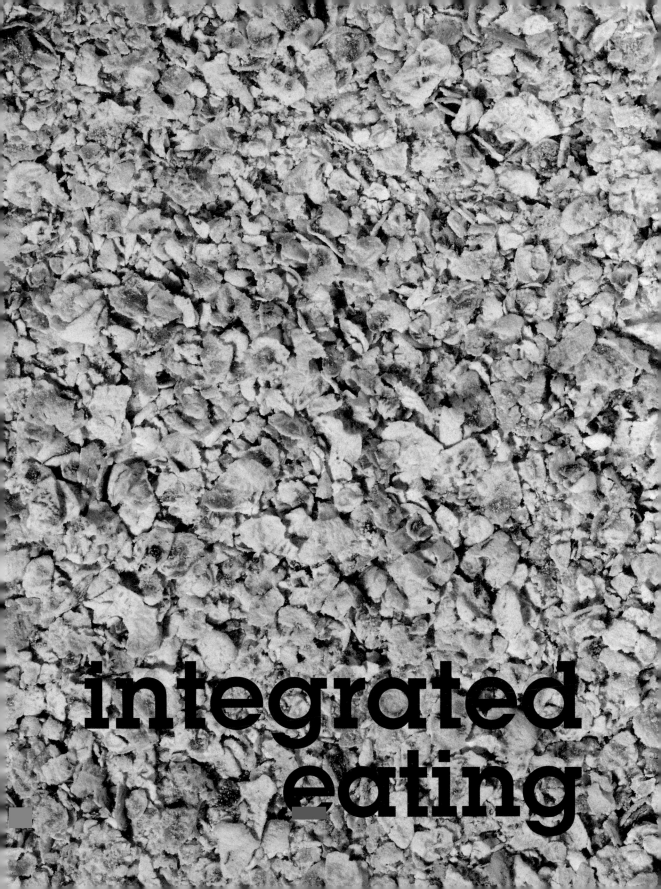

integrated
eating

fuel for life

A healthy eating plan boils down to consuming the right sorts of foods in the right quantities to provide enough energy to sustain your body through whatever level of activity you choose to do. The trick is not to lose your way in today's ever-growing dietary maze.

Perhaps the most crucial thing to remember when adopting changes to the way you eat is to make sure that you create a diet that you can enjoy. A common mistake among failed dieters is to stock up on foods they think they should be eating; then, when it comes to the crunch and they are ravenously hungry, a mung bean salad is not that appealing so they end up ordering in a high-fat pepperoni pizza instead.

In this chapter I will introduce some nutritional basics, giving you sufficient knowledge to formulate a dietary regime that will supplement and support your integrated exercise plan. I will also outline some of the pitfalls associated with food shopping and help you to play supermarket detective in the hope of avoiding them. The idea is to stock your freezer, fridge and store cupboard with quick-to-prepare foods that are wholesome but which will also satisfy your appetite and of course your taste buds. You need to adopt a healthier eating plan gradually, rather than making drastic changes overnight, and ensure that it is one which you feel comfortable enough with to stick to over the long term.

work it out

Nibbling on **cheese and crackers** may seem like a healthier option than gobbling down a box of chocolates, but the calories do still mount up. A small, matchbox size, chunk of blue cheese such as Stilton provides 102 calories (there are 114 in Cheddar). Add even the lowest-calorie crispbread (17 calories) or a cream cracker (35 calories) and you'd have to do one of the following to work off those calories:

- work out intensely to a celebrity fitness video for 20 minutes
- wash up and put away dishes after a festive spread for 34 minutes
- fill bags with rubbish, bottles and newspapers to take to the recycling centre for 30 minutes
- battle your way through busy shops for 28 minutes
- prepare sandwiches, tea and cakes, then wash up for unexpected guests for 38 minutes
- play board games for 48 minutes.

Just how much fuel do you need?

How many calories you need to consume in order to maintain, lose or gain weight is dependent on your individual Basal Metabolic Rate (or BMR). The BMR is a minimum requirement – that is, the number of calories the body needs just to stay alive, including those burned for essential functions such as heart rate, brain activity and breathing.

In someone who is inactive the BMR can represent up to 75 per cent of their total energy expenditure, but the more exercise they do, the more calories their body burns in excess of its BMR. Physiologists have developed a number of ways in which to calculate the BMR; of these, the Harris-Benedict, devised in the 1940s, is considered one of the most accurate. Here's how to calculate it:

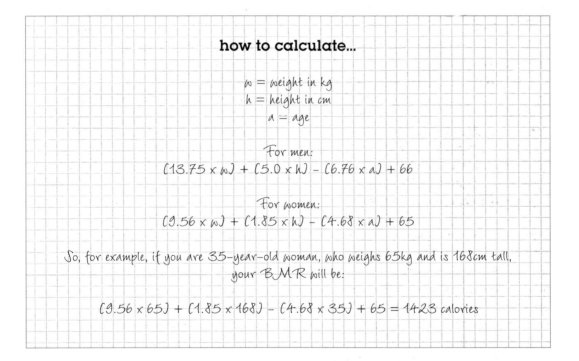

how to calculate...

w = weight in kg
h = height in cm
a = age

For men:
$(13.75 \times w) + (5.0 \times h) - (6.76 \times a) + 66$

For women:
$(9.56 \times w) + (1.85 \times h) - (4.68 \times a) + 65$

So, for example, if you are 35-year-old woman, who weighs 65kg and is 168cm tall, your BMR will be:

$(9.56 \times 65) + (1.85 \times 168) - (4.68 \times 35) + 65 = 1423$ calories

Next, to calculate the number of calories you need to maintain your current weight, you multiply your BMR by the following amounts according to your levels of activity:

Sedentary – you do very little exercise and have a job that requires you to sit down for most of the day: BMR x 1.4

Quite active – you are fairly active throughout the day and make a conscious effort not to sit down all the time: BMR x 1.7

Very active – you play a lot of sport or have a very physically demanding job: BMR x 2.0

how to lose weight and keep it off

Start by assessing your current diet. It is only when you can see clearly what you are doing wrong that you can set about making it right. Keep a record of all your food and fluid intake for at least a three-day period (including one weekend day). You should try to be as honest with yourself as possible.

Calculate your daily calorie aim. Using the formula above, work out your BMR and then your individual energy needs to see how many calories you require to maintain your current weight. Next, subtract 15–20 per cent from this total to determine your daily calorie aim. Cut out convenience, fast and processed foods and fatty snacks. These usually contain a lot of refined sugar, are bad news for your body and will cause energy slumps, leaving you more prone to snacking. Many processed foods also lack nutrients, so try and replace them with more nutritious and less calorific, low-GI (see page 151) snacks that will fill you up.

Don't skip meals. In fact, the key to healthy eating is to eat little and often rather than consuming three large meals a day. This will prevent the drop in blood-sugar levels that so often triggers a corresponding dip in energy levels, resulting in bingeing on unhealthy snacks.

Don't starve. Cutting calories too drastically increases the production of the stress hormone cortisol and insulin, which controls blood-sugar levels. Consequently, the body responds by storing excess calories in the abdominal region. Mostly the calories are stored as fat which is why otherwise very thin people can still have a roly-poly belly.

Get in your daily fruit and veg quota. An intake of at least five portions of fruit and vegetables a day has been found to ward off cancer, heart disease and other major killers. It shouldn't be difficult to achieve – fresh, frozen, chilled, canned, dried and juice all count towards the total – yet most of us fail to meet the daily target. One portion of fruit is, for example, half a large grapefruit, a slice of melon or two satsumas. A glass of 100 per cent juice (fruit or vegetable) counts as a portion, but you can only count one glass a day, however much you drink, because it provides very little fibre. One portion of vegetables is equal to three tablespoonfuls of cooked carrots or peas, or one cereal bowl of mixed salad. As a starchy food, potatoes don't count.

Plan ahead. Do you have a habit of eating on the run? Or do the time and place of your meal affect your food choices? Do you rely heavily on takeaway meals? Maybe you eat differently at work, for example, because there are limited options available. Get into the habit of planning ahead to make sure you aren't caught short on the nutrient front. Gradually gain control of your diet and you will notice big changes in the way you feel and look.

dietary essentials

Contrary to what many faddy diets suggest, a healthy eating plan must incorporate energy from three different fuel sources in food – fats, protein and carbohydrates. Too much of any of them can be unhealthy, as can too little. What is important is getting the balance right.

Fat

Despite what you may hear, fat should not be cut out of your diet completely. In fact, some fat is needed to function healthily; problems only arise when we consume too much fat. The current health recommendation is to get no more than 35 per cent of your total calorie intake from fat and less than 10 per cent of all calories should be from saturated fat. However, ideally your total fat intake should be somewhere in the region of 20–25 per cent of the calories you consume. Here is a guide to help you navigate your way around fats and fatty acids:

Trans-fatty acids

These are a particular kind of fat produced when plant-based oils are 'hydrogenated' to produce solid spreads, such as margarines. They're often found in confectionery and processed foods including pastry, biscuits and cakes. Trans-fatty acids have been found to have the same effect on cholesterol levels as saturated fat and should be avoided as much as possible.

Saturated fats

These are mainly derived from animal sources, such as the fat found in meat and in dairy products such as butter and cheese. It is also found in coconut oil and palm oil. Too much saturated fat has been linked to a higher risk of heart disease and so intake should be limited.

Polyunsaturated fats

These have been separated by scientists into omega-3 and omega-6 essential fatty acids (EFAs). Neither of these is produced by the body but both are needed to keep us healthy. It is, therefore, crucial to include them in your diet. Good sources of omega-3s (derived from linolenic acid) are rapeseed, evening primrose and walnut oils, although the richest supply is in fish oils. It is recommended we consume two portions a week of fish, including one of oily fish such as mackerel, herring or tuna. Half a pint a day of organic milk gives you a useful additional supply, and a matchbox-sized pieced of organic cheese will provide you with 88 per cent of your (recommended daily intake) RDI of linolenic acid. Omega-6s (derived from linoleic acid) are found in most edible oils (particularly sunflower and corn) and in meat.

Monounsaturated fats

These fats – considered to be the healthiest type – are thought to protect against heart disease. They are found in olive oil, peanuts and avocados. A Mediterranean diet, which is rich in fruit, vegetables and monounsaturated fats (usually olive oil) is believed to extend life expectancy.

Protein

Every cell in the body needs protein to function – it is also important for helping muscles, bones, hair and fingernails to grow. Protein in food is broken down through digestive enzymes into amino acids which are absorbed by the body and used to make more protein. There are twenty different amino acids found in plant and animal food, most of which can be made by the body. However there are eight 'essential' amino acids that cannot be produced naturally and have to be obtained through diet. While studies have shown protein to be useful in any weight-loss plan, too much is bad news; a high-protein diet can also be high in fat and put unnecessary strain on the liver and kidneys. It is recommended that around 15 per cent of your total calories come from low-fat protein foods.

Carbohydrates

Carbohydrates have received bad press in recent years, partly through diets such as the Atkins and the Zone which advocated limiting carbohydrate intake to an absolute minimum. However, very low-carbohydrate/high-protein diets have been proven to have some unhealthy side effects (ranging from headaches, bad breath and constipation to an increased risk of heart disease) and are not necessarily a safe route to weight loss.

In fact, some carbohydrate foods are essential for well-being and are especially important in a more active lifestyle. There are two main groups of carbohydrates, grouped according to their chemical structure – 'simple' sugars (sucrose, fructose, glucose and highly processed sweet foods) and 'complex' starches and fibres (potatoes, bread, pasta and rice).

Carbohydrates are the muscles' favourite source of fuel to help them perform any type of activity (from walking to ironing). However, the body has only a limited capacity for storing them (as glycogen in the muscles and a little as glucose in the bloodstream) which means they must be consumed regularly. If levels are not constantly topped up, the result is extreme fatigue and light-headedness.

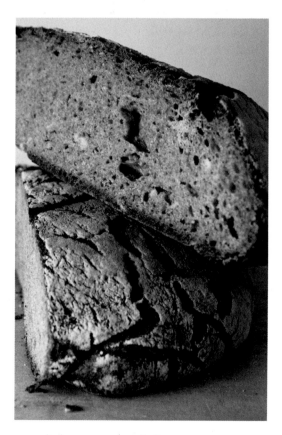

The glycaemic index (GI)

While starchy carbohydrates provide fibre and a long-lasting energy boost, there is another way of determining which carbohydrates are most helpful in the diet. The glycaemic index (or GI) is a ranking system based on the rate at which different foods raise blood-sugar levels.

Foods with a low GI rating release sugars into the body more slowly and evenly, leaving you feeling full. High-GI foods, on the other hand, such as cakes, white bread, biscuits and highly processed foods cause blood sugar to soar and then crash, sometimes triggering a cycle of hunger, snacking and weight gain. A predominantly low-GI diet, on the other hand, is a potentially healthier way of eating all round, incorporating foods that are higher in fibre, lower in sugar and less processed.

Getting used to GI ratings and their effects on your body can take a little time and experimentation, although some food labels do now include a GI score to help consumers. The table below gives examples of foods that have high, medium and low GI ratings; remember that while all carbohydrate foods are important energy suppliers, the best have a low GI.

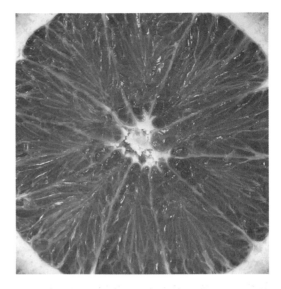

did you know?

Studies have shown that eating a low-GI breakfast of muesli, porridge or wholegrain bread leads to less snacking between meals and to considerably fewer calories being eaten at lunchtime, even when subjects were offered an all-you-can-eat buffet!

High-GI foods	Medium-GI foods	Low-GI foods
Baked potato	Pitta bread	Lentils
Honey	Brown rice	Oranges
Sports drinks	Muesli bars	Spaghetti
White bread	Pineapple	Bananas
Watermelon	Melon	Baked beans
Sweets (e.g. jelly babies)	Raisins	Oats
French stick	Carrots	Apples
White rice	New potatoes (boiled)	Dried apricots
Parsnips	Ice cream	Peanuts

Vitamins and minerals

If you include a wide enough variety of foods in your diet you should not need expensive nutritional supplements to obtain them.

Vitamin A is needed to help the body's cells grow and develop as well as to improve vision and immune function. It comes in two forms: retinol in animal foods and beta carotene in fruit and vegetables. Vitamin A obtained from plant sources has important antioxidants that help to ward off disease. RDI (Reference Daily Intake): 700mcg (men); 600 mcg (women).

Vitamin B1 (thiamin) enables the body to get energy from carbohydrates and fats. It also prevents the build-up of toxic substances in the body. RDI: 1mg (men); 0.8mg (women).

Vitamin B2 (riboflavin) releases energy from food to enable vitamin B6 to function properly. RDI: 1.3mg (men); 1.1mg (women).

Vitamin B6 (pyridoxine) is vital for the formation of oxygen-carrying red blood cells (too little can result in a form of anaemia). It is also important for good immune function and the release of energy from protein-rich foods. RDI: 1.4mg (men); 1.2mg (women).

Vitamin B12 (cynacobalamin) is crucial for making DNA and myelin – the sheath that surrounds the body's nerve fibes. RDI: 1.5mcg (men); 1.5mcg (women).

Vitamin C (ascorbic acid) is a disease-fighting antioxidant that also helps the body to absorb iron from food. It is needed to produce collagen (a protein essential for healthy bones, teeth, skin, cartilage and gums). RDI: 40mg (men and women; smokers need at least 80mg a day as the habit destroys vitamin C).

Vitamin D (calciferols) is needed to absorb the calcium and phosphorous required for the formation of bones and teeth. RDI: exposure to daylight should be enough (at least 20 minutes a day), but if this isn't possible you need around 10mcg a day from food.

Vitamin E is an antioxidant that helps to prevent damaging free radical substances from harming cell membranes and other tissues. RDI: at least 4mg (men) and 3mg (women).

Folic acid is needed to form DNA and essential proteins in the body. RDI: 200mcg (men and women); 400mcg during pregnancy.

Calcium ensures the healthy growth of bones and teeth and is essential for muscle function. RDI: 700mg (men and women).

Magnesium is important for the growth of bones and teeth and helps to ensure that nerve impulses function well. RDI: 300mg (men); 270mg (women).

Potassium helps to maintain the balance of body salts (electrolytes) in the body and to keep heartbeat and blood pressure at healthy levels. RDI: 3500mg a day (men and women).

Iron is essential for the formation of red blood cells and a large number of the enzymes involved in energy metabolism. RDI: 8.7mg (men); 14.5mg (women).

Selenium is an antioxidant mineral that protects against infection and free radical damage. RDI: 75mcg (men); 60mcg (women).

Zinc is vital for fertility, reproductive function and development. RDI: 9.5mg (men); 7mg (women).

Food sources for vitamins

Vitamin A : Egg yolks, Cheese, Oily fish (e.g. sardines, salmon), Liver, Green leafy vegetables, Carrots, Butternut squash, Apricots, Cantaloupe melon

Vitamin B1: Fortified bread and breakfast cereals, Offal, Pork, Potatoes, Nuts, Pulses

Vitamin B2: Dairy foods, Eggs, Meat, Fish, Fortified breakfast cereals

Vitamin B6: Lean meat, Poultry, Fish, Wholemeal bread and cereals, Bananas, Nuts, Soya beans

Vitamin B12: Meat, Fish, Eggs, Dairy foods

Vitamin C: Fresh fruit and vegetables (including juices), especially strawberries, blueberries, kiwi fruit, blackcurrants, oranges

Vitamin D: Fish oil, Eggs, Fortified margarines, Oily fish

Vitamin E: Nuts, Seeds, Vegetable oils, Fortified margarines

Folic acid: Leafy green vegetables, Liver, Brussels sprouts, Pulses, Wholewheat bread, Fortified breakfast cereals

Food sources for minerals

Calcium: Dairy foods (best source), Leafy green vegetables, Tinned sardines (with bones), Sesame seeds

Magnesium: Wholegrain cereals, Nuts, Seeds, Green vegetables, Pulses

Potassium: Bananas, Citrus fruits, Avocados, Dried fruit

Iron: Offal, Sardines, Egg yolks, Dark green vegetables, Fortified cereals

Selenium: Meat, Fish, Dairy foods, Brazil nuts, Avocados, Lentils

Zinc: Oysters and seafood, Red meat, Peanuts, Sunflower seeds

food labelling

Food labels are becoming increasingly detailed which can be useful but also confusing if you are not familiar with the terminology. Beware of the following phrases:

- Flavour/flavoured: a food described this way may not contain the ingredient it is flavoured with. So, cheese and onion flavoured crisps need not contain cheese or onions.

- Fresh, pure and natural: there is no legal definition for these terms.

- Extra fruit: if a label makes this claim, it must list the total amount of fruit the product contains.

- Fat-free: no legal definition.

- Light/lite: no legal definition.

- Reduced salt/sodium: no legal definition.

- No added sugar: no legal definition (and products can be sweetened in other ways with syrups, honey or fructose).

- Unsweetened: no legal definition.

Is it healthy?

How do you tell if a food is too high or low in sugar, fat or salt? Look carefully at how many grams of each there is for every 100g of a product then use the following guide to assess its health merits:

High	Low
20g or more fat	3g or less fat
5g or more saturated fat	1g or less saturated fat
0.5g sodium	0.1g sodium
10g total sugars	2g total sugars

---

did you know?

The target for salt intake is no more than 6 grams a day, yet on average we consume twice that amount.

- Too much salt is linked to high blood pressure and an increased risk of heart disease. It is also thought to affect demineralisation of bones which could raise the risk of osteoporosis.

- Around 75 per cent of the salt we eat is added by manufacturers with foods such as bread, some breakfast cereals and ready meals being the worst offenders. Only 10 per cent occurs naturally and 15 per cent is added at the table or in cooking.

drink to your health

Staying hydrated by drinking regularly is vital to health. Fluid is required by every cell in the body and a failure to drink enough will leave you feeling tired and lacking in concentration and can affect the way you look and feel. In general, the advice is to consume around 2 litres (or 8 cups) of fluid every day. This does not have to be water – tea, coffee, fruit juice and even soup can count towards your daily tally. The more activity you do and the hotter the weather, the more fluid you will need.

But it may be surprising to learn that you can actually drink too much. Hyponatraemia – a condition caused by water toxicity whereby the levels of body salts in the bloodstream become dangerously dilute – is becoming increasingly common, especially among those who lead active lifestyles.

So how much is it safe to sip? Precise amounts vary according to body size and weather conditions, but aiming to consume no more than a litre of fluid for every hour of activity will maintain a healthy fluid balance. A simple way to ensure you replace losses is to weigh yourself before and after vigorous or prolonged exercise – for every pound you lose, you will need around two medium glasses of water to replenish fluid levels.

A word on alcohol

Enjoy a tipple? Well, even though you are embarking on a healthier way of life there is no need to give up alcohol altogether. Plenty of evidence shows that a glass of wine (most favour red wine, although white also has purported benefits) is rich in antioxidants and helps to ward off heart disease. The key is not to overdo it. Medical recommendations for alcohol consumption are 14 units a week for women and 21 for men (one unit being the equivalent of half a glass of beer or a small glass of wine).

If you regularly over-indulge, your risk of cardiovascular disease rises as does the likelihood of high blood pressure. A high intake in women is also linked to a greater risk of breast cancer and lowered fertility. In addition, it can also influence your appearance – the nutrient supply to your hair, skin and nails is affected if you drink too much too often and you must, of course, also watch the calories (a glass of white wine contains 85; a pint of beer has 170). Drinking a few small glasses a week, however, is not thought to be harmful.

ten (surprising) eating-for-fitness tips

1 **Have a steak and eggs:** A protein-rich diet is thought to help weight loss when combined with exercise because it contains a high level of the amino acid leucine which stimulates muscle synthesis and recovery.

2 **Suck a mint:** Psychologists asked 40 athletes to run hard for 15 minutes on a treadmill while inhaling one of four scents – peppermint, jasmine, dimethyl or a non-odour control. Those who inhaled peppermint perceived themselves to be making less effort and could, therefore, keep running for longer. The minty scent probably enhances breathing by clearing the airways.

3 **Pump up on iron:** More than one-third of women don't get their daily iron requirement (14.5mg) from recommended iron-rich foods such as red meat, chicken, eggs, leafy green vegetables and fortified cereals. And too little iron can make getting fit an uphill struggle.

4 **Get your oats:** Tests on a wide range of different foods grouped according to their GI rating found porridge (made with oats and water) to provide the longest-lasting energy boost when eaten prior to a workout. Porridge-eating athletes performed even better than those who took a high-tech energy sports drink.

5 **Eat tinned peaches:** Sports nutritionists confirmed tinned peaches to be fitness friendly. Research showed that athletes given a low-GI meal of tinned peaches and muesli performed better in a 60-minute run 3 hours later than those who had been given a high-GI breakfast.

6 **Nibble on nuts:** All nuts are a rich source of dietary protein that is needed to enhance the recovery of muscles after intense exercise, but cashews (unsalted) are particularly effective. They also contain carbohydrate and essential minerals like potassium (lost in sweat), so they are particularly useful after a workout. A 50g serving of cashews, for example, provides one-fifth of a woman's daily iron requirement.

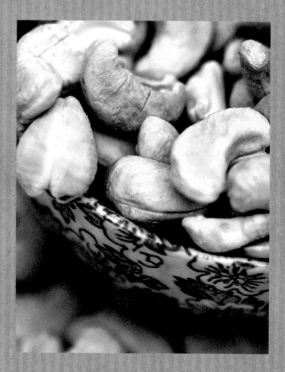

7 **Drink flat cola:** Researchers at the Australian Institute of Sport (AIS) in Canberra have found that sipping 1–2 cups of either flat cola (the non-diet variety) or black coffee can boost your endurance capabilities by up to 3 per cent. Cyclists who sipped on the beverages before and during exercise were able to keep pedalling for longer and faster than those who took plain water. It also helps you to burn fat. However, remember that too much caffeine (in excess of six cups a day) has been linked to less healthy side effects, so restrict your daily intake.

8 **Eat breakfast:** Breakfasts kick-starts your metabolism which becomes sluggish overnight and, as such, is the most important meal of the day. A daily breakast of cereal and toast also helps to stave off mid-morning cravings for fatty snacks, thereby helping to keep weight in check.

9 **Avoid chewing gum:** Researchers have found that chewing gum makes you swallow a lot of air which inflates the belly until it is expelled. Smokers and fast talkers experience the same problem.

10 **Drink milk:** Don't waste money on expensive energy drinks. Chocolate-flavoured milk has been shown to help boost recovery after exercise as effectively as any commercial sports drinks. US researchers have also discovered that a glass of semi-skimmed milk post-workout speeds up fat burning and encourages faster muscle gain.

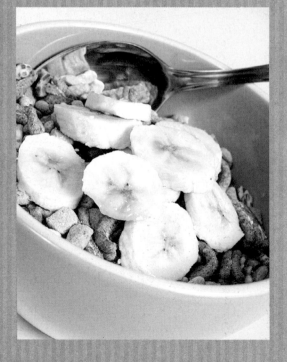

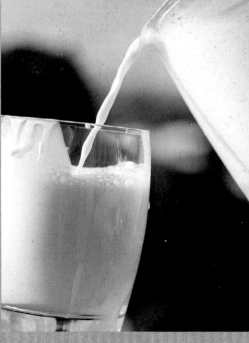

index

resources

Gear and Gadgets

Babyjoggers and fitness strollers

www.kidsense.co.uk (tel. 0116 2751895) or www.babyrunner.com (01844 278314).

Bambach saddle seats

For information go to www.bambach.co.uk or call 0800 581108.

Footwear

Crocs

Brightly coloured, rubbery, waterproof clogs that are good for people with foot-health problems. Go to www.crocsfootwear.co.uk for details of stockists.

Fitflops

Wedged flip-flops that allegedly 'destabilise' the foot to make leg, bottom and stomach muscles work harder. Go to www.fitflop.com for details.

MBTs

Shoes that have been shown to help reduce arthritic and back pain in some people. Go to www.mbt-uk.com or call 020 7684 4633 for more information.

Heelys

Trainers with either one or two wheels in the heels. For details visit www.heelys.com.

Fitness

Cycling

Contact the charity Sustrans (www.sustrans.org.uk; tel. 08415 113 0065) for details of the 10,000 miles of paths on the Network or join the Cyclists Touring Club (www.ctc.org.uk; tel. 0870 873 0060) which organises group rides and events for all levels.

Dancing

For details of dancing and other activities, contact the Central Council for Physical Recreation (CCPR): ccpr.org.uk (tel. 020 7976 3900).

In-line skating

For information about in-line skating courses in the UK and abroad: citiskate.co.uk; tel 020 7228 2999.

Mall walking

Several shopping centres in the UK now hold mall-walking sessions including the following:

Leeds White Rose Shopping Centre (www.white-rose.co.uk), Birmingham Bull Ring (www.bullring.co.uk), Manchester Trafford Centre (www.traffordcentre.co.uk)

Nordic walking

Information on Nordic walking classes, technique and suppliers of poles: nordicwalking.co.uk (tel. 020 8878 8108).

Pushchair workout classes

Classes are held in the UK, Europe as well as the USA. For details, go to www.buggyfit.co.uk (or call 01844 202 081), www.strollerstrides.com or www.strollerfit.com.

Running

Ukathletics.net (tel. 0121 713 8400) or runnersworld.co.uk for information about running.

Skipping

For details of qualified skipping coaches for workshops, go to www.skipping-workshops.co.uk (tel. 020 8786 7707) or www.skip2bfit.co.uk (tel. 01843 603020).

Tree climbing

Information about tree climbing courses and general advice in the UK: mighty-oak.co.uk (tel. 07890 698 651).

Walking

Walking the Way to Health (whi.org.uk; tel. 01242 533337) is a joint initiative between Natural England and the British Heart Foundation that supports over 400 local walking schemes. Includes details of the National Stepometer Programme.

General Health

British Nutrition Foundation

For information about healthy eating and weight loss: www.nutrition.org.uk (tel. 020 7404 6504)

British Heart Foundation

For details of 30 a day and other campaigns: www.bhf.org.uk (tel. 020 7935 0185).

Chartered Society of Physiotherapy

For advice and tips on healthy gardening: csp.org.uk (tel. 020 7306 6666).

National Osteoporosis Society

nos.org.uk (tel: 0845 130 3076) for information about how exercise can build strong bones.